Auditory Training
for Deaf Mutism
and Acquired Deafness

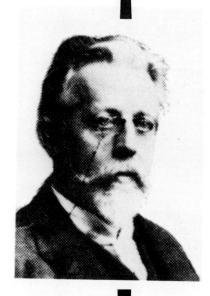

Victor Urbantschitsch

Auditory Training for Deaf Mutism and Acquired Deafness *by Victor Urbantschitsch, Royal and Imperial Professor of Otology at the University, and Chairman of the Section of Ear Diseases of the General Polyclinic in Vienna, Austria is a classic in the field. This work was originally published in German in 1895 by the publishing house of Urban & Schwarzenberg in Vienna and has been translated in 1981 by Dr. S. Richard Silverman, Director Emeritus of the Central Institute for the Deaf and Professor of Audiology, Washington University, St. Louis, Missouri.*

Auditory Training

for Deaf Mutism

and Acquired Deafness

Victor Urbantschitsch

translated by

S. Richard Silverman, Ph.D.

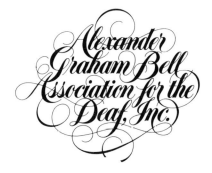

Alexander Graham Bell
Association for the Deaf
3417 Volta Place, N.W.
Washington, D.C. 20007

Library of Congress Cataloging in Publication Data

Auditory Training for Deaf Mutism and Acquired Deafness Urbantschitsch, Victor-Silverman, S. Richard, translator

Library of Congress Catalogue Card Number 82–70281

ISBN 0–88200–151–5

© 1982 by the Alexander Graham Bell Association for the Deaf

3417 Volta Place, N.W.

Washington, D.C. 20007

Printed in the United States of America

10   9   8   7   6   5   4   3   2   1

Acknowledgment

The Alexander Graham Bell Association for the Deaf is honored to publish this valuable landmark in the history of oral education. We would also like to recognize Dr. S. Richard Silverman's admirable devotion to this notable task, encouraged by Dr. George Fellendorf, formerly Executive Director of the Association and Dr. Brigitta Hauger, of Georgetown University, for her additional expertise in technical translation.

Translator's Preface

   This translation of Victor Urbantschitsch's *Hörübugen bei Taubstummheit und bei Ertaubung im Späteren Lebensalter* was stimulated by the growing scientific and professional interest in the possibilities of improving the education of hearing-impaired children through what is now generally termed auditory training. It is my considered judgement, that however they may vary in details of technique and procedure, current rationales and practices all in some way have been influenced by the work of Urbantschitsch. That we are unaware of his seminal contribution may be due, not as much to indifference to what is foreign or to preoccupation with what is contemporary, as to the unavailability of the original material in our own language. Consequently, the primary aim of the translation is to make available in English Urbantschitsch's theorizing, observations, procedures and disputations on auditory training, and a wide range of related topics as he, himself expressed them. I wish to make it emphatically clear that in so doing, neither defense, criticism, or espousal of Urbantschitsch's text is intended. These judgements are left to the reader.

   Victor Urbantschitsch (1847–1921) was appointed the first head of the Department of Otology of the internationally renowned Vienna Otolaryngological Clinic in 1872. His investigations in the anatomy and function of the Eustachian tube laid the foundation for improved therapeutic procedures involving the tube and the middle ear. But the consuming passion of his entire professional career appeared to be "otological acoustics." In fact, Prof. E.H. Majer, himself a former professor at the Polyclinic, suggests in his notes on the history of otolaryngology in Austria that "based on his many pertinent works Urbantschitsch can be called the father of audiology." (1980).[1] (In his *History of the International Association of Logopedics and Phoniatrics* Perello assigns this encomium to Friedrich Bezold (1976).)[2] It is interesting to note here that, in the main, leadership in modern continental audiology is vested in individuals who bring to it medical training in otology. In 1907, Urbantschitsch, by then Professor, was named to succeed the legendary Adam Politzer as Director of the Vienna University Otological Clinic. Urbantschitsch's book on Otology, *Lehrbuch der Ohrenheilkunde*, had by 1910 been put out in its fifth edition. He was also editor of the journal *Monatsschrift fur Ohrenheilkunde*.

The present volume intended as a treatise devoted exclusively to auditory training, as its title indicates, touches on an impressive number of topics that can be properly labeled audiological. Included among them are entries dealing with auditory fatigue, central versus peripheral deafness, binaural hearing, tactile perception, effects of noise, emotional impact of hearing impairment, influence of hearing impairment on acquisition of speech and language and on employment, "adult" rehabilitation, auditory sequels to diseases such as meningitis, syphilis and scarlatina, transfer of training, training of personnel, and motivation to submit to rigorous training regimes. These are incorporated into the exposition by a predominantly clinical case-cum-theorizing method. Although Urbantschitsch's critics would more than likely have deprecated his theorizing on some of these matters, and considered them unsound and unfounded, if not wild, speculations, they did recognize that they came within the clinician's purview as worthy of attention and study. He was more of an originator than an instrument of the times.

The central point of Urbantschitsch's argument is that the education and ultimately the emotional and social adjustment of profoundly deaf children could be facilitated by methodical and persistent auditory training (exercises) that exploited any remnant of residual hearing by stimulating what he termed a dormant auditory sense. Although auditory training was not an entirely novel idea, as Urbantschitsch was quick to state (note his references), his stubborn insistence on its value, his diligence in producing objective supportive evidence, and his theoretical rationalization of his particular approach attracted a considerable amount of professional attention from medical colleagues and educators of the deaf never evidenced before that time. The reaction was mixed, leaning more toward skepticism, if not downright opposition, than to approval and acceptance—a pattern that was to be repeated in America. Even the great Politzer tended to denigrate Urbantschitsch's work.

Prominent among those who shared Urbantschitsch's interest in auditory training was Friederich Bezold, Professor of Otology at the University of Munich, who worked with deaf children at the Munich Central Institute for Deaf Mutes as Urbantschitsch worked with pupils at the Döbling Institute for the Deaf, located in the outskirts of Vienna. Bezold based his training on careful analysis of specific "tonal defects and islands," described in detail in his *Das Hörvermögen der Taubstummen* (1896)[3] and directed his structured training to them while Urbantschitsch, also exceedingly analytical and methodical in his approach, stressed the need to arouse (*erwecken*) a dormant state of areas even where residual hearing was not at first evident, including total (*vollständig*) deafness. Urbantschitsch believed, so to speak, that there was more there than initially meets the ear. In contrast to Urbantschitsch's initial use of concertina-generated tones and single vowels, Bezold emphasized larger speech input units for training. He rejected Urbantschitsch's notion that physical hearing or the "efficiency of the acoustic nerve" could be improved by training.

Although Bezold's views and procedures appeared to gain more acceptance than those of Urbantschitsch, the latter never wavered in his convictions and enthusiasm. Perhaps, given present day skepticism about the "cost benefits" of auditory training for profoundly deaf children, Urbantschitsch's perseverance and resolve may constitute more of a legacy than his rationale and his method. I had the good fortune to experience lively and provocative exposure to these attitudes in my studies and association with the late Dr. Max A. Goldstein from 1933 until his death in 1941. As part of his post-graduate studies at the Vienna clinic in 1893, Goldstein worked with Urbantschitsch and was so impressed and stimulated by his mentor's work with deaf children that he joined him in daily training sessions with the children at the Döbling Institute. Urbantschitsch was equally impressed by his young colleague's capability and enthusiasm and subsequently exhorted him to introduce his method to America and to convince all who would listen that congenitally deaf children could, by his approach, learn to talk intelligibly. This experience as much as anything moved Goldstein to found the Central Institute for the Deaf in St. Louis in 1914 and to complement a distinguished career of medical practice, education and leadership with a sustained devotion to the improvement of the education of hearing-impaired children.

Translation of literature of a scientific or professional specialty requires of the translator not only a working knowledge of the language but most importantly it demands reasonable experience, if not thorough expertness, in the area under consideration. Generic terms take on very specific and exclusive meanings in the context of specialty lexicons and discourse. Here and there the precise intent of the original writer may be unclear to the translator especially if the vintage of the literature is of another era in the development of the subject. This is the case in the present translation. For example, there may be some question about what Urbantschitsch intended in the use of such terms as *Wahrnehmung, Empfindung, Perception* and *Verstandnis*. These could represent the progression from awareness to sensation to perception to comprehension not to mention concepts such as detection, identification, discrimination, recognition and cognition. Yet in a general linguistic sense the meanings of the German words may very well overlap or be synonymous. I mention in passing that the most frequently occurring of the above German words in the text is *Empfindung*. I have generally favored *sensation* as the translation for this word. I have taken my cue from the conventional translation of Helmholtz's classic *Tonempfindungen*, published in 1863. Urbantschitsch cites Helmholtz and was undoubtedly influenced by his work.

My interpretation of the writer's intent in questionable places in the text has been guided by careful consideration of the particular contexts in which they occur. I have consulted knowledgeable colleagues about puzzling items but, any errors of interpretation or of accuracy are, of course, solely mine.

Acknowledgments

I acknowledge gratefully the loan of the original German text by Professor Dr. Milos Sovak, Prague CSSR, and express my thanks to Dr. George W. Fellendorf, former Executive Director of the Alexander Graham Bell Association for the Deaf, who arranged the loan and duplication of the text. I am indebted to Professor Emeritus, Dr. E.H. Majer of the Ear, Nose and Throat Department of the Vienna Polyclinic for the biographical material on Victor Urbantschitsch. To my colleague Dr. Ruediger R. Thalmann, Professor of Otolaryngology at Washington University, who at one time was associated with the Vienna Polyclinic, goes my appreciation for easing me over an occasional rough spot in the translation. The encouragement of Dr. Donald R. Calvert, Director of Central Institute for the Deaf, has been very helpful. As important as any contribution to the performance of my task has been the understanding support and durable patience of my wife, Sally, who put up with the not infrequent undulations of mood growing out of my encounters with Urbantschitsch's prose. The willingness of these individuals to help in this enterprise reinforces my conviction that the gift of professional maturity is more likely to come to those who know the history of their field.

It is not without sentiment that I offer this translation. My experience in its accomplishment has made me realize more than ever how deeply indebted I am to those who have preceded us for their noteworthy contributions, their exemplary diligence and their unshakable conviction in the value for deaf persons of communication by speech. And in a very special sense I shall be forever grateful to Prof. Victor Urbantschitsch's student, Dr. Max Aaron Goldstein, my teacher, to whose memory this rewarding labor is appreciatively and affectionately dedicated.

S. Richard Silverman
St. Louis, Missouri
June, 1981

Foreword

Victor Urbantschitsch

In the following essay I present an expanded treatment of the lectures which I delivered at the General Polyclinic in Vienna during the academic year 1894–95 concerning the effect on the sense of hearing of systematic auditory training. Because of the growing interest in this subject I hope a more detailed presentation of the material will call the basic significance of hearing exercises to the attention of a wider circle.

As noted in the course, systematic auditory training demands complete dedication and unrelenting patience. What better goal for humanitarian and didactic efforts could there be, than the quickening of a dormant sensory function? Who would not feel richly rewarded in his efforts in finding an opportunity to prove to himself the value of awakening the sense of hearing, even in a case of apparent total deafness, or in seeing the salutary effects on the psyche, on the mental processes, and on the social life of a deaf patient that auditory training can have!

If only from the humanitarian standpoint, there is abundant compensation in applying diligent effort to develop the auditory sense. But the interest is just as great from the scientific standpoint. Here is a substantial area for psycho-physiological investigation, both in research into early manifestations of hearing, as well as in a variety of related phenomena that accompany the maturation of the sense of hearing. In communicating my observations concerning this work I am acutely aware that many gaps remain and that further thorough research has yet to yield many valuable findings.

In communicating first about findings dealing with manifestations of individual deaf and deafened persons, I have included a general discussion of relevant psycho-physiological observations and pathological findings, even if these did not deal particularly with the deaf mutes and the deaf. I have done this in order to present a clear exposition of current knowledge of the phenomena concerned. To a large extent, I have made use of my own papers which appeared in *Pflüger's* "Archiv der Physiologie" in the "Archiv der Ohrenheilkunde" and in *Schwartze's* "Handbuch der Ohrenheilkunde" and which I will refer to when indicated. Excerpts are included without disrupting the continuity of presentation of the main topic.

With regard to polemically expressed positions to be found in these papers, I emphasize explicitly that I was not moved by personal motives but only by the cause which I espouse. I certainly value all opinions if they are based on expert knowledge and are documented by one's own practical experience. However, under certain circumstances I deem it necessary to oppose purely theoretical reasoning and opinions which contradict facts, especially in subject matter which is accessible only by experience, like auditory training. Simple discussion is, to be sure, easy, but effective participation requires a great deal of effort. Should my advocacy be judged rather trenchant, it should be kept in mind that every attack on an undertaking that is still in its initial stages can be all the more dangerous if it comes from a respected source. For this reason, I deem it necessary to defend myself vigorously. I repeat that I am guided only by strictly factual standards and not by personal motives, but that I feel obligated to represent the cause itself in a decisive and forceful manner.

Even if later, more thorough studies of auditory training may correct some judgments rendered in this paper or even if they are completely repudiated, it is of no consequence to the cause itself. I ask only that the subject be thoroughly examined from a great many sides. From the humanitarian standpoint, I consider it impossible ever to abandon a method of treatment, which, even if it cannot heal, can often relieve the sad condition of the congenitally deaf and persons with acquired deafness. It is my heartfelt conviction that general application of auditory training will lead to its general acceptance. I would consider myself generously rewarded if this treatise can contribute a little to this cause.

Urbantschitsch
August, 1895

Contents

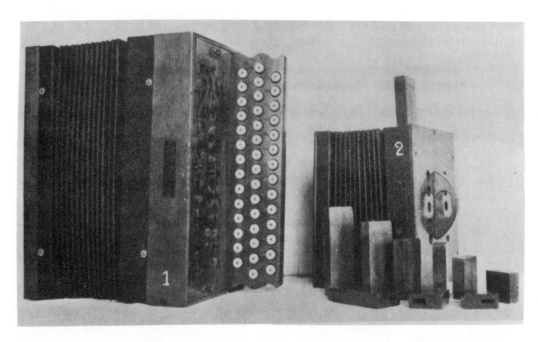

1—Goldstein's accordion (concertina) with keyboard of six octave range, eight notes to each octave. 2—Urbantschitsch harmonika (concertina) with individual reeds. (From Goldstein, M.A., *The Acoustic Method for the Training of the Deaf and Hard-of-Hearing Child*. St. Louis, Mo.: Laryngoscope Press, 1939, p. 25.)

Introduction

In presenting an exclusive discussion on the effect of systematic auditory training on the sense of hearing, I hope that in the course of this effort my treatment does not appear to be unjustified and that the great significance that I attribute to such training is not considered to be exaggerated.

Before I get into the specifics of systematic auditory training, I should like to discuss its practical value from a general point of view. The attack on hearing impairment is directed primarily and basically against the diseases of the conducting or of the sensing parts of the auditory mechanism. On the one hand we can postulate one class of hearing loss in which a normal functioning sense organ receives impulses which are too weak; on the other hand, another class where sufficiently intense stimulation cannot exert a proportionate effect on the diseased organ. Furthermore, both of these conditions can occur together, or a lesion originally limited to the conductive apparatus can produce a gradual diminution of hearing because of weak stimulation of sensory activity.

Causes of hearing impairment

Taking these phenomena into account, therapeutic efforts have been aimed at affecting a perhaps defective sound conduction or at increasing the diminished auditory function. In the latter connection, it has been shown that till now, the attempts have been frequently more or less ineffective. Still, they are sometimes successful if the di-

Management of involvement of the acoustic nerve

minished auditory responsiveness is associated with a general illness, the improvement or elimination of which has a beneficial effect on the organ of hearing. More rarely though is it effective on an exclusively circumscribed involvement of the acoustic nerve. Thus, localized maneuvering primarily with electrotherapy unfortunately does not often achieve the desired result. How often we come across cases where hearing impairment increases despite a variety of therapeutic measures and all kinds of attempts to help! Is there still a possibility for improvement in these cases? Is there some other way that acoustic capability can be stimulated directly besides the conventional methods that have been applied till now? Familiar to us, indeed, is the great influence of massage and body gymnastics in involvements of muscle and nerve. From this the idea follows that in many cases easing of conductive or perceptual difficulties through stimulation of the involved sense organ primarily employing auditory gymnastics can possibly improve the inadequately functioning and even the defective organ.

Auditory gymnastics

It is an obvious assumption that among all possible stimuli the auditory nerve can be excited most intensively by means of acoustic stimuli. The soundness of this assumption has been increasingly validated in the course of my investigations and I hope in my presentation to show convincingly the diverse and important effectiveness of systematic auditory training.

The effect of systematic auditory training on the sense of hearing can be shown for congenital deafness as well as for acquired hearing impairment or deafness. Although the acoustic management of both of these groups is essentially the same, it is expedient from a practical point of view to discuss auditory training for deaf mutes and for those who became deaf later in life separately. I shall first consider the acoustic training of the deaf.

Chapter One

The Effect of Systematic Auditory Training on the Sense of Hearing in the Deaf

Historical Review

The notion of influencing the sense of hearing of the deaf through auditory training is an old one indeed. Already *Archigenes*[4] in the first century A.D. mentioned the hearing tube and intense sound as method for stimulating a weakened sense of hearing, as did *Alexander of Tralles*[5] in the sixth century; *Guido Guidi* (1595)[6] recommended arousal and training of latent hearing by noise and shouting.

*Ernaud** in 1761 reported a new method by which deaf persons were enabled to discriminate tones. This con-

---

*Academy of Science of Paris, 22 January 1761; see *Boyer*, La Voix, Paris, 1895, Vi, Nr. 61 for detailed references to French publications on auditory training for the deaf. In this article *Boyer* seems to assume that in my reports concerning results of auditory training with the deaf I have not given due credit to French authors, which could give the impression that I had been the first one to be active in this field. That such an interpretation is not warranted is well documented by my first report on the subject (Wiener Klin. Wochenschr., July, 1893, Nr. 29) which begins with the following words: "The idea of improving the auditory capability of the deaf by means of auditory training is not at all new." Furthermore, in this and later publications I have clearly emphasized the credit due *Itard* for his work in this field. (Wiener Klin. Wochenschr., January, 1894, Nr. 1; paper presented at the scientific congress in Vienna, September, 1894).

cerned deaf people, however, who could hear phonemes, if only indistinctly, and who were trained to progress to hearing words. In a more specifically reported case Ernaud achieved hearing for sentences. Of interest is *Ernaud's* assertion that absolute deafness does not occur, and also his judgment of the questionable value of a hearing tube for training. Seven years later *Péreire*[7] reported his observations that almost all the deaf could attain hearing for words if they were not totally deaf. *Péreire* used a hearing tube for his exercises.

Itard[8] was the first to carry on basic investigations of deaf mutes, particularly the study of the potential effect of auditory training on deafness. This distinguished observer noted in his research, first undertaken in 1802, that many deaf persons could improve their perception of sound through continuous input of sound to the ear. In 1805 he began extensive tests with six deaf mutes. *Itard* commenced the lessons with a bell and gradually reduced its intensity in the course of instruction; then followed various musical tones, rhythmic drum beats, after this, tones sounded by a flute, later the five vowels and finally the consonants. The lessons were subsequently continued with only three deaf subjects who throughout one year received a daily lesson of one hour. The final results follow: One of the three subjects who had originally heard only thunder and tones of the bell achieved hearing of words; the second, who had better original hearing than the first pupil, experienced a much more significant improvement in hearing; the third deaf mute, however, the most gifted of the three pupils, whose original hearing was comparatively the best, showed significant hearing progress only at the beginning and finally finished behind the other two because he just did not relish the exhausting drills.

The auditory training introduced by *Itard* was continued by *Valade-Gabel*[9] and after *Itard's* death in 1838, by *Blanchet*[10] who used speech and various musical instruments. Also, at this time *Deleau*[11] spoke encouragingly about auditory training for the deaf. Other noteworthy promising results were observed by *Piroux*[10], in Nancy, and by teachers at the institute for the deaf in Bern.[11]

In Germany in the first half of this century, increasing numbers of writers advocated auditory training for the deaf.

Beck[12] proposes the following:

The sounds themselves must be used to stimulate the diminished function of the auditory nerve and to rouse it out of its inactivity. Vibrating tones are the best stimuli for the ear, as they are essential for sensory activation. We can then employ musical instruments which produce rushing tones; we can beat a drum closer or farther depending on the level of deafness; we can accomplish stimulation of the auditory nerve of hearing by striking a bell sometimes louder and sometimes more softly. This procedure must be initiated in the case of deaf mutes whose deafness is not total (*Itard*).

Jäger[13] likewise achieved results by auditory training of the deaf. *Wolff** described an extremely valuable method for "orthophonic and orthoacoustic" instruction by which a deaf child can be taught speech and hearing of vowels and consonants simultaneously. *Frank*[14] comments that a residual amount of auditory sensitivity in the deaf should be enhanced as much as possible by training, more specifically several times a day by bells, drums and whistles, after which planned auditory instruction takes the place of these sounds.

Toynbee[15], in London, emphasizes the possibility of improvement in those deaf who can already hear vowels. He reports three cases concerning two deaf persons who experienced significant improvement in hearing through systematic training; in the third case, a 70-year-old man who had lost his hearing many years previously was stimulated by systematic auditory training to such a degree that he could communicate by a hearing tube with various people.

In France, interest in auditory training subsequently waned more and more.[16] But more recently, in North America, increasing attention has been paid to the subject.

Lincke, Handbuch der Ohrenheilkunde, 1845, III, p. 223, in p. 262–268 of the same volume reference is made to the Spanish, Italian, English, French and Latin literature on the deaf and their education.

Gallaudet in 1884 introduced two deaf persons for whom systematic auditory training had yielded encouraging results. Since then auditory training for the partially deaf has been instituted in various schools for the deaf in North America, among which *Currier* in New York and *Gillespie* in Nebraska are especially outstanding. In recent years, a committee in the U.S.A. made up of *Graham Bell, Gordon* and *Clarke* met and in its report recommended highly the investigations of *Itard* and recommended extensive research in auditory training. Such investigations are likely to be instituted presently in many schools in North America. In 1894, a committee under the chairmanship of *Gillespie* was organized to work for the spreading of auditory training.

Stimulated by results attained in North America, *Javal*[17] in Paris (1888) suggested the establishment of special classes for auditory training where partially deaf mute persons would be instructed on an experimental basis. *Dufo de Germane* reported on this in a paper in 1892.[17]

Systematic auditory training for the deaf is currently being used in Bourg la Reine near Paris. This includes the use of a hearing tube constructed by *Verrier* by which reportedly favorable results were attained. Investigations were carried on with these tubes in various institutes for the deaf including some in Austria. Nevertheless these attempts were soon abandoned.

Despite all the many-faceted and repeated attempts and despite many noteworthy individual results achieved systematic auditory training has till now not been generally undertaken. Instead, schools for the deaf in various countries have limited themselves to recommending rather than employing auditory training, mostly in cases where residual hearing, especially for vowels, could be demonstrated. As has been demonstrated for the last 25 years by Director Lehfeld among others[18], some very striking hearing results were achieved in individual cases where there was hearing for vowels. As a matter of fact, *Lehfeld* emphasizes that in the phonetics class every teacher of the deaf exploit every bit of their residual hearing, which is frequently enhanced by these exercises. After termination of this program, however, exercises are usually discontinued, and the result is a regression of the improvement attained. Within recent years, I have met with teachers of the deaf and deaf persons in various institutes both at home and abroad and besides have made many inquiries concerning efforts in auditory training. My experience has always been the same, namely, that acoustic exercises even in cases of obvious substantial residual hearing are generally completely neglected except in isolated cases and, furthermore, are almost never practiced with children who apparently are either totally or nearly deaf. Various papers on deaf mutes and the education of the deaf, including recent ones, represent a distressing picture, all in all, of the almost inconceivable neglect of the organ of hearing of the deaf in general.

In 1888 and 1889, I achieved an improvement in hearing of a deaf boy through two years of continued systematic auditory training which amazed me at that time. In the beginning the boy was able to hear only single sounds spoken loudly in his ear but in the course of making use of his auditory training gradually was able to hear sentences spoken at moderate volume one to two paces from his ear. Finally he was able to pursue a regular school curriculum. This observation caused me to pay more attention to auditory training for the deaf and especially since 1892, I have become acquainted with the results of systematic auditory training for a steadily increasing number of the deaf. This gave me a great deal of satisfaction. There were among these deaf people cases which I, along with the prevailing opinion of colleagues in our speciality, in the past years would have thought not able to hear and unsuited for anything but an exclusive training for deaf mutes. Nevertheless they not only acquired perception for vowels, but gradually were able to hear complete sentences. Initial tests in many of these cases indicated apparent total deafness so that there was perception neither for dissimilar tuning fork tones, presented to the head or by air conduction, nor for vowels shouted loudly into the ear even with assistance from a hearing aid.

The reception accorded my first reports convinced

*Opinions about the
value of auditory
training*

me that the significance of auditory training in general
and particularly in the apparently totally deaf was not only
completely unknown before then among experts in various
countries, but even doubted or denied.[19]

I was taken to task on the grounds that the time and
energy spent on the training were not consistent with the
attainable results.[20] At the third congress of German teachers of the deaf in Augsburg (May, 1894) *Director Hemmes*
gave a lecture favoring acoustic training and commented
therein that evaluations of my auditory training by experts
from institutes for the deaf sounded with few exceptions
"unfavorable, disapproving, and cool."[21] *Hönigmann*[22] recommends the adoption of a wait-and-see position all the
more so because two well-known Viennese otologists were
unfavorably inclined.

At the same time, I must give even more prominent
recognition to the Lower Austria State School for the Deaf
in Döbling-Vienna where *Professor Lustkandl* has shown an
active interest in instituting experimental acoustic training
and where, in addition, *Director Lehfeld* and Instructor of
the Deaf *Kühnel* along with the other active teachers have
undertaken auditory training with great dedication and
perseverance. They created some justified excitement and
experienced general acceptance by their impressive dem-
onstration of trained pupils before the Medical Society of
Vienna on 1 December, 1893, on 27 April 1894, and at
the congress of natural scientists in Vienna on 27 September 1894.

The individuals in these schools who began experiments with 60 pupils have presented evidence that aural
instruction for the deaf can show results not only in isolated
cases, but that it can be successful also in schools including
children who were believed to be totally deaf.

Also *Hemmes*[23] in his previously mentioned lecture says,
"Experiments continued over an extended period with
children who were judged to be hopelessly deaf, have convinced me that with them, too, hearing results are attainable." *Hemmes* consequently agrees completely with the
statement that I had published ten months before.[24] Six
months before *Hemmes'* lecture, *Bestic*,[25] stimulated by the

positive results in Vienna, reported that he had instituted systematic auditory training with favorable outcomes in the school for the deaf in Agram.

The Volta Bureau in Washington showed a special interest in these auditory training procedures and, as I learned through personal communication, experiments in systematic auditory training were introduced in a few schools for the deaf in North America, including work with apparently totally deaf mute persons.[26] Also, these acoustic exercises were sympathetically received at the congress of natural scientists in Vienna (September, 1894), and by this time several otologists are employing auditory training. In addition, I welcome with great pleasure increasing indications of a more active interest in systematic auditory training on the part of various teachers of the deaf, since for the deaf this training can be a great boon if teachers of the deaf accept it, and if it becomes a required subject in schools for the deaf. A very significant step in this direction was taken by the Lower Austrian Diet at its session on 1 February 1895. Acting on a report by a member of the regional Diet, *Nicholas Dumba*, who expressed his satisfaction at the introduction and results of systematic auditory training in the State School for the Deaf in Döbling, the Diet immediately authorized the Lower Austrian Board to support this training.

To be sure, it will take a long time before the systematic auditory training introduced in the Döbling School for the Deaf will achieve a breakthrough; as long as the success achieved thus far in Vienna continues to be subjected from various quarters to the familiar pattern of being totally ignored or of being characterized as insignificant or as old hat. In the most recent handbook on the education of the deaf by *Walther*[27] we find on page 73 the following statement: "In modern times almost all institutes for the deaf have undertaken systematic auditory training." In this connection, *Walther* cites the presentation by *Hemmes* and states further: "Up till now the results are still very negligible."

It is worth noting that *Walther* draws only on the presentation by *Hemmes* and ignores the reports emanating from Vienna. It is, however, true that at the Augsburg

Congress of Teachers of the Deaf (May, 1894), the Viennese efforts were by no means favorably recognized and previously published reports were not held worth mentioning, despite the fact that the comments by *Hemmes* could only confirm these reports. Furthermore, *Walther* also ignores the publicly demonstrated results of systematic auditory training with the pupils of the Döbling School for the Deaf before the scientific congress in Vienna in September, 1894. This attitude does indeed appear strange because in such an important humanitarian concern as the acoustic training of the deaf undoubtedly is, it appears totally irrelevant whether renewed efforts emanate from Vienna, Augsburg, or Berlin. Instead, every success story coming from a reliable source should at least be worthy of an investigation or deserve a reference in a Handbook for the Education of the Deaf, if for no other reason than that it could lead to further encouragement of such investigations by unbiased readers. In this case we have expected this all the more, since Walther, probably based on his own experience with results of auditory training, felt justified in claiming: "Up till now the results are still very negligible," while the Döbling School has demonstrated very significant results which can easily convince anyone and which in fact have convinced an ever increasing number of expert visitors, thanks to the congenial cooperation of the director and teachers of that institution. In all of this, the Döbling School for the Deaf is just beginning its efforts in systematic hearing instruction and still has many difficulties to overcome until the acoustic curriculum will be directed on an orderly course and attain the high level that we all have in mind.

Walther's statement that in recent times "almost all institutes for the deaf have undertaken systematic auditory training" would, indeed, be welcome, but it does not agree with recent reports that have come to me from various sources. Perhaps such instruction is given on a more private basis and only to individual deaf students and the majority of the deaf are not involved. But even conceding that such systematic auditory training is really universally practiced in almost all schools for the deaf, there appears to be a great difference in the method of implementation when compared with that of the Döbling School where the outcomes, as previously mentioned, have already been shown to be significant and are still improving while *Walther* still terms the results he knows negligible.

With the introduction of systematic auditory training in schools for the deaf and its application to those with apparent total deafness, a new and demanding professional teaching specialty is emerging requiring total dedication, sacrifice and unflagging patience. I am nevertheless convinced that the teachers of the deaf, whose beneficial work we cannot, in any event, praise enough, will make this sacrifice for the well being of their pupils. When we acquire insight into the difficulty of this kind of auditory training we become aware of the magnitude of their effort. But in the end, those who hold a negative view of these auditory exercises either because of doubt or indifference, should just once witness the intense impression which the awakening of a new sense evokes in the deaf, the joy, the surprise or deep emotion (the latter particularly with the adult deaf) when for the first time they experience distinct hearing and understanding of speech. They should observe how enthusiastically the pupils at the school for the deaf enter into the exercises and how left out they feel when lack of time keeps them from being included in the training. They should all learn to know more specifically the favorable influence that successful auditory training has on the lugubrious spirit of the deaf, when the improvement in hearing gradually lessens the feeling of isolation which pervades many a deaf person, who sees himself cut off from his fellow human beings in so many ways because of his misfortune. When we observe the powerful influence on the psychological development of the deaf resulting from improvement of hearing by acoustic exercises and, moreover, when we are convinced by the advantages which will be documented below that accrue to the deaf depending on the level of the achieved improvement, then all opposition and doubt as well as indifference to the value of systematic auditory training must wane. And taking for granted that all of us have a sympathetic feeling for the misfortune of the deaf, I am convinced that everyone will ultimately declare his support for systematic auditory training.

This would constitute a true source of blessing, considering the lamentable condition of the deaf. Even if only a small number profits from it, the lot of many of these unfortunates would be improved. Just consider that in Europe alone, there are 200,000 deaf mutes, and about 40,000 in the United States of North America.

Undertaking systematic auditory training

I now turn to a discussion of systematic auditory training itself and start with a description of the method that I use. If I describe this method in great detail, I do so because in the beginning of my investigations, in cases of apparent total deafness I felt the lack of a practical method for stimulating auditory responsiveness. At least I did not come upon any relevant precise information, but was referred to the mostly aphoristic remarks which I have cited above in my historical review. The reason may lie in the fact that auditory training, at least as far as I can see from the reports concerned, was limited to the deaf with partial hearing, especially to those children described as half deaf and that the so-called totally deaf, with rare exceptions (see, for example, *Itard*) were not included. However, the arousal of a completely dormant sense of hearing requires a distinctive method. Of course, training of partial residual hearing likewise requires patience and perseverance but the method is actually self-evident and requires no detailed description, especially since an exemplary guide to "orthophonic and orthoacoustic" exercises by *Wolff*[28] is available, according to which single sounds can be learned phonetically and acoustically at the same time.

Over the years, I became increasingly convinced that much depends on the method itself in the more difficult cases. Time and time again cases were presented to me with the judgment that all hearing tests with them had foundered and consequently there was no prospect of good results. Yet the method of auditory training described here led to results which were encouraging, and what is more, in certain cases, surprisingly favorable. I am sure, of course, that there are several deficiencies in this method and that wider experience as well as a good deal of individualization of it will lead to substantial change and expansion.

Description of the Method

I now posit the case of apparently total or nearly total deafness, a case where at initial examination, different tuning fork tones and especially the powerful sounds from a concertina as well as single vowels shouted directly into the ear yield only a negligible or no impression of hearing.

I begin the training by speaking a loud and sustained vowel, usually / a / or / o: / repeatedly into the ear of the deaf person who already understands through lipreading. In case this does not give rise to auditory perception, I make the same attempt with another vowel. If these attempts yield no result, I repeat them with increased intensity accomplished by shaping a funnel with the hollow of both hands through which I speak into the ear. I hardly ever use speaking tubes for this because they affect the quality of the voice significantly while this is not the case when a soft-surfaced sound funnel is shaped by the hands. Frequently the first signs of hearing appear with this procedure using intensified sounds; if, however, there is still no such response, then I stimulate the ear for a longer time with a concertina tone corresponding to one of the training vowels, usually for several minutes. One advantage of using the concertina is its greater penetrating power as compared to the human voice, another is that this procedure affords a rest for the person who has to administer the training and urgently needs some respite during the longer exercises. In this connection I should like to point out that these acoustic lessons place a great demand on the physical strength of the teacher and that a weak constitution is generally not sufficient to administer them.

Speech sounds

A concertina I had made especially for the purpose of testing and exercising hearing proved to be particularly useful. Tones on a scale of 6 octaves (E^{-1} to e^4) can be set on it either singly or, for the purpose of training of discrimination, also in pairs. Pressure on the big air chamber

Concertina tones

can activate these tones continuously and very strongly or softly, whatever is desired. A manometer fixed to the air chamber can indicate differences of 1/10,000–1/10 of atmospheric pressure and allows measurement of the tone intensities which are easily adjustable by varying strength of pressure on the air chamber. In this way a measure of hearing sensitivity is available. This concertina enables me to test the hearing capability for each single tone and to train an initially weak or totally absent acoustic excitability for particular tones. Particularly in the latter connection the concertina will prove to be especially useful to the training of hearing because it can produce a specific intensity of tone which surpasses that of tuning forks considerably. It can therefore indicate that some forms of deafness demonstrated by tuning forks are not true deafness but only an especially low excitability for the hearing sensations involved. For auditory instruction in schools for the deaf, the concertina as well as the harmonium (reed organ) serve a valuable function.* With these instruments, auditory training can be carried out for several children simultaneously. At the present time at the Döbling School for the Deaf, there are a number of concertinas in daily use in individual classes and are preferred for use by teachers engaged in auditory instruction, particularly in the early development of audition.

As evidence for the suitability of concertina tones in acoustic drills, I offer an observation made with a deaf person who initially understood various vowels spoken into the ear only after I had previously got her to react to related tones of the concertina until she heard them clearly corresponding to those vowels spoken by my voice. Many other cases convinced me that striking improvement in hearing for speech can be achieved by instruction with the harmonium or concertina tones, a fact which is also very important for the purpose of self-instruction.

Binaural sound stimulation

In those rather rare cases where strong and repeated stimulation by tones did not arouse the slightest trace of hearing, I was occasionally successful in eliciting initial au-

---

* As I subsequently learned *Roller* recommended the Concertina for auditory purposes. (Deutsche Naturforscher-Versammlung, 1884)

ditory sensations by presenting sounds simultaneously to both ears; this happened every time in a case when the sound in question was presented through a T-shaped tube simultaneously to both ears where activation of hearing could not be elicited through the left or right ear alone. A patient who could not perceive a loudly presented / a / either on the right or left side always did so in each ear when the / a / was shouted simultaneously by two persons into both ears. I made the same observation when a vowel acted intensely on one ear and a corresponding concertina tone on the other. At the same time, both ears could still show dissimilar characteristics. In a 22 year old deaf person who after repeated lessons was gradually able to discriminate / e: /, / I / and / o: / in the right ear and who showed only the slightest trace of hearing in the left ear, I tried to get a response for / a /. Despite speaking / a / loudly into his right or left ear, many such exercises did not yield the slightest sensation of sound nor did my simultaneous presentation of a loud concertina tone corresponding to / a / to the better hearing right ear and a spoken / a / to the worse-hearing left ear. On the other hand, a reversal of the procedure always yielded a more or less significant hearing response by the otherwise poorer-hearing left ear when while speaking an / a / in the left ear a powerful concertina tone was presented to the right ear. By control tests I satisfied myself that it was not a question of the auditory sensation of concertina tones influencing the left ear inasmuch as every sensation disappeared at the moment when presentation of / a / in the left ear was interrupted during presentation of a continuous concertina tone. Occasionally, an increase in hearing can be elicited when two unrelated stimuli are introduced—one to the right, the other to the left ear, leading to acoustic recognition of one or both of the stimuli. Thus one of the deaf recognized the word *Lampe* (lamp) in the right ear when some word, for example *Fenster* (window), *Polster* (cushion) was simultaneously presented to the left ear; with simultaneous presentation of the word *Lampe* in the right and left ear this word was repeatedly heard simultaneously in both ears while otherwise each ear was unable to do so individually.

Frequently acoustic activation that has been achieved

Gradual acoustic fading

by binaural sound stimulation can be demonstrated even some time after the sound has faded; thus immediately after a binaural sound stimulation monaural auditory responsiveness is sometimes possible over an individually varying period of time but usually only for a few seconds— an indication that the heightened wave of auditory excitement recedes only gradually.

Binaural hearing

I have already reported detailed investigations concerning hearing function of monaural versus binaural hearing.[29] My interpretation of the increased hearing function accompanying binaural hearing was as follows: added to the auditory impulse reaching each ear externally, there is another centrally located subjective impulse which is caused by the effect of the stimulated acoustic center of one side on that of the other. At the same time, my investigations suggested to me that when in one ear sensitivity is still below the threshold, stimulation of that ear can have an effect on the acoustic center of the other. Consequently, in the case of binaural hearing, the better hearing ear can be assisted by the other ear even when the hearing in that ear is somewhat below threshold. Assistance to the better hearing ear from the poorer one by no means requires the same sound to operate on both ears but the effect is also achieved when both ears are subjected to dissimilar acoustic stimuli, which I was able to show in acoustic training of the deaf, confirming my previous investigations.[30] Although adequate sound presentation to both ears may affect mostly the mutual functional activity, the just mentioned results show that even the poorer-hearing ear can help in achieving greater acoustic arousal in the other better ear generally as long as there is any trace of hearing left in the poorer ear. Similarly in the case of binocular vision one eye can experience improved sight as long as the other eye is at all sensitive to light, even if that eye, owing to an anomaly of refraction, is not by itself able to perceive an object.[31]

By continuing attempts of this kind, a permanent increase in acoustic excitability is gradually attainable, until finally sound stimulation of one ear only can elicit an auditory response in that ear. At this point systematic auditory training for the person concerned can be continued in the normal way.

Again, in another situation the first trace of hearing can be observed only after prolonged sound stimulation and thus we frequently find deafness or particularly poor hearing ability in the beginning of a training session which improves visibly in the course of the lesson. An otherwise familiar word spoken into the ear for the first time is often not heard before it has been repeated several times. A formerly totally deaf man who gradually attained his hearing through auditory training told me that when speaking loudly to himself he could hear nothing initially but after a few minutes he could hear single phonemes, then syllables, after a while words and finally whole sentences.

Continuous sound stimulation

Through the exercises, which in the majority of cases are fortunately not always that laborious and lengthy, the deaf mute achieves an ever increasing hearing impression with a particular vowel called into the ear; however, in cases of initial vowel deafness, the vowel concerned is not yet recognized, e.g. / a / as "a"; the subject achieves this only later with the acquisition of discriminatory hearing.

Arousing first traces of hearing

As soon as specific hearing is indicated for one vowel we should proceed to practice with another vowel until it, too, elicits a hearing impression. At this stage, there is the feasibility of beginning the training of discrimination hearing. To this end, the two vowels are now repeatedly spoken slowly and clearly into the ear in a sequence known to the deaf person. In this way he or she gradually gets to know the difference in hearing which results from comparing acoustic stimuli and, in the course of further instruction, is increasingly able to recognize single vowels aurally. However, in this case, too frequent drilling is usually necessary in order to fix the proper auditory perception. It is common that vowels previously heard correctly are confused with one another or that a particular vowel repeatedly spoken into the ear gives the hearing impression of different vowels. When, for example, drills with the vowels / a /, / I /, / o / have been given and these vowels could already be auditorily clearly differentiated and correctly repeated, confusion appears in subsequent drills, or when

Training for discrimination

/ a / is spoken into the ear three times in succession the response is / a /, / I /, / o /. As additional vowels and subsequently consonants are included in the auditory training, errors in auditory discrimination appear more frequently and their elimination demands the greatest patience and perseverance. Whenever such confusions occur I strongly recommend that the incorrectly identified sound and the one that has actually been presented be repeated one after another in order that the difference clearly emerges. Phonemes that are difficult to recognize must especially be practiced and also those that are easily confused, / b / and / p /, / d / and / t /, / b / and / d /, / g / and / k /.

In this connection, there are noticeable individual differences. Particular phonemes are clearly perceived by some deaf individuals in a short time, by others only after many weeks or even months of training. This is also the case for such speech sounds which usually present little difficulty. Thus, even / a / may elicit an incorrect response or none at all in a situation of an otherwise already advanced state of hearing where, for example, the other vowels and even consonants are clearly discriminated. Frequently there are difficulties in hearing the difference between / e / and / I / or for one of these vowels in isolation. Thus, in one case, for example, despite four weeks of training / e / was not heard at all and / I / was identified as / a / and only by further auditory training did the responsiveness to both of these vowels gradually increase. In another case, weeks of training were necessary before / a / and / e / were not heard as / I / but were correctly heard individually.

These experiences already indicate that training in auditory discrimination of single speech sounds requires very laborious and lengthy instruction. Thus there is the very possible danger that especially children's interest in these lessons may decrease to a point where they take part in them only unwillingly.

Importance of motivating auditory training

It is, therefore, very important from the pedagogical standpoint to establish motivation for auditory training as soon as possible. This is usually accomplished if we go on to easily understood words as soon as just a few vowels and consonants can be recognized. For this, it is best to begin with practice of auditory discrimination of simple words which are meaningful such as *Mama, Papa,* and *Auge* (eye), *Nase* (nose), etc. Here the appropriate word is initially communicated to the deaf person in advance, because a word presented to the ear for the first time is not recognized even if the deaf mute is able to hear the speech sounds of this word individually. Further practice of different words is carried out just as with various speech sounds. The auditory impression stimulated by repeated speaking of a particular word leads to an auditory image of the word which the otherwise speech-deaf person is able to recognize among many still unfamiliar auditory sensations. In this way, an ever increasing number of words can be drilled on* just as in the learning of a foreign language, and auditory discrimination can be developed even at a stage where auditory capability is still very limited in general.

Auditory images

Short sentences can also be practiced in this way and after frequent repetition are recognized more and more easily. This acoustic memorizing becomes an important means for the acquisition of a vocabulary and even, as has already been mentioned, in a situation of prevailing deafness for speech where a person is not able to hear unfamiliar words, not even single syllables, and still shows great deficiency in the discrimination of vowels.

In this connection, it is of great interest to trace the gradual emergence of such auditory images while we speak a sentence or a word familiar from previous drills slowly and with clear enunciation repeatedly into the ear of the deaf person. The first response can be completely incorrect; it may not even concern similar sounding words, but for the most part words which have already been repeated in earlier lessons. Only after frequent repetition of these words will they be partially or completely understood. I present here only a few examples: A deaf mute girl who

---

* For each deaf person who undertakes such training I maintain a notebook in which the practiced words are entered; in so doing, it is recommended that the well understood words are underlined in order to know the easily recognized discriminable cues of those words compared to those of the difficult ones. In simultaneous training of both ears the right page of such a notebook can be designated for the right ear, the left page for the left one. In this way we get a convenient overview of the words easily understood in each ear.

previously had responded correctly and repeatedly to the two sentences *Die Grille zirpt* (the cricket chirps) and *Die Mühle klappert* (the mill clatters), the first time understood *Die Grille zirpt* as *Die Mühle klappert*, right after that as *Die Grille klappert*, and then heard it correctly the third time as *Die Grille zirpt*. A man, nearly deaf to speech perceived the sentence *Heute ist es trüb* (Today it is overcast) as *Lampe* (lamp), *Fenster* (window), *trüb* (cloudy) since in the course of preceding lessons the words *Lampe* and *Fenster* had become familiar to him. The sentence *Wie geht es Ihnen?* (How are you?) was heard as *Heute ist es trüb*, in another case only as / a / and / o /, the word *Fenster* repeatedly articulated was identified as *Fenster* but the second time as *Lampe*, thus, strangely enough, correct for the first time but incorrectly heard the second time, immediately following, an observation that is often made. The sentence *Der Bauer pflügt* (The farmer plows) was understood by a deaf person as *Lampe, Nase*; the next day the same person heard several words and short sentences correctly either immediately at the first presentation or, at least, when they were repeated into his ear.

More frequent are confusions of similar sounding words, or, in the case of frequently practiced words or sentences, singly heard words or syllables are used as cues for the combination of words or whole sentences. I select, for example, the sentences: *Der Bauer pflügt, die Grille zirpt*. When the subject to be trained repeats these sentences familiar to him correctly several times, that does not prove that every syllable was actually heard. Thus, in one case only the / a / from the first sentence and just the / I / from the second was perceived, which led to a correct combination of both sentences. Obviously this is even easier if individual syllables from previously presented familiar sentences are perceived. That this is more a combining or synthesizing action rather than actual hearing is shown by incorrect responses when the words of the two sentences are interchanged or the word order reversed. In the case when both sentences *Der Bauer pflügt, die Grille zirpt* are correctly repeated the sentence *Der Bauer zirpt* (the farmer chirps) or *Die Grille pflügt* (the cricket plows) is at first

Auditory combination

usually incorrectly repeated; thus the person in training gets the word *zirpt* then this gets combined with the other words *die Grille* or the word *pflügt* with *der Bauer*. For this reason in the presentation of sentences, word order is of the greatest importance. It should be emphasized to the student that nonsensical sentences are given and that he needs to depend only on his ear and not on combining. I also do this frequently in drills on single words in which, for example, I omit the initial sound or some other sound of the drill word so that the word makes no sense.

In the course of ongoing training words should be selected that are difficult to discriminate from one another such as *Wand* (wall), *Sand* (sand), *Tand* (trifles), *Land* (land), *Pfand** (pledge), etc. This discrimination usually presents greater difficulties than the comprehension of sentences. It is often striking how spectacularly well and easily many persons are able to understand sentences and entire conversations who exhibit very limited auditory discrimination when tested more precisely. Indeed, I have carried on entire conversations with several people who absolutely could not hear some sounds or syllables, among them syllables of a word that the persons consistently repeated correctly. Therefore one should never neglect exercises with sounds and syllables which are difficult to understand, as well as with similar sounding words. One part of an acoustic training session should always be reserved for the refinement of auditory discrimination.

Using similar sounding words and sounds

Auditory Training for Children in the First Years of Life

For deaf or severely hard-of-hearing children in the first years of life musical tones, above all, lend themselves to the awakening of the auditory sense, especially those of the concertina, which should be played into the ears frequently during the day. However, in the case of an un-

---

* For this purpose there is a very good selection of such words in the work of *Roderich Benedix, Die deutliche Aussprache* (Distinct Articulation) Part I; this also includes a compilation of especially difficult words and sentences.

pleasantly strong reaction an appropriate softening of the tone is strictly called for; suitable, in addition, are the various wind and string instruments, music boxes commonly used as toys, wind-up toys, and bells as well as any devices which produce distinctive sounds. With children beginning at ages two or three I recommend, in addition, the introduction of auditory speech lessons repeatedly during the day, initially by showing the child an object, e.g. in a picture book, and simultaneously calling the appropriate word into the ear. In this way auditory images are created, the importance of which I have stressed previously. Later these can occasionally lead to auditory comprehension of short sentences. From age five on, orthophonic and orthoacoustic exercises can begin and auditory training by the method described above can be instituted.

Sound Intensity

The strength of an auditory sensation depends, as I have previously demonstrated, not only on intensity per se but also on the duration of the pertinent signal[32]. Thus, given equal intensity, a hearing response can sometimes occur and fail to occur at other times depending on whether the sound stimulus was short or prolonged. Hence, a sound spoken loudly into the ear will frequently generate no impression of hearing if presented once for a brief time while the same sound spoken less intensely but prolonged for a long time can result in a significant auditory sensation. Therefore, in auditory training, the proper intensity and duration of the auditory stimulus must be carefully taken into account.

Regarding the sound intensity itself, it is especially important that only that level be used which appears to be absolutely necessary to stimulate an auditory response.

In my experience a too powerful sound stimulus giving rise to an especially intense acoustic stimulus produces an early auditory fatigue that is harmful and irritating instead of stimulating. A severely hard-of-hearing person reported to me that shouting into his ear for a few seconds produced a notable improvement in hearing followed by a considerable persistent hearing impairment for a prolonged period of time. To produce a positive effect on hearing function, the sound should have only so much intensity that a certain attentiveness is required to hear it. How auditory exercises undertaken in this way stimulate hearing ability can be very clearly seen in its occasionally quite significant increase during such instruction.[33]

It is quite common that words or sentences which on first presentation are either not heard or are heard incorrectly are ever more clearly perceived after repeated presentation without raising the voice. One patient who had to undertake self-instruction by means of loud platform speaking at first heard only a confusing noise when using a steady volume but after a minute heard single sounds, then syllables, words and, only after a few minutes, whole sentences.

Similarly, as in the case of exercises using speech, we must also be on guard against excessive intensity of sound in training with musical tones as, for example, with tones of the concertina. Thus here, too, in every individual case we should establish the sound stimulation absolutely necessary to activate auditory response and, in so doing, we should pay attention to the often variable sensitivity to sound depending on pitch. In many cases, the tone intensity required for a high-pitched tone, for example, is likely to be quite different and frequently much higher than that for a low-pitched tone. In case that even the most intense tone stimulus that can be produced with the appropriate instrument, as with the concertina, still does not result in any indication of hearing, then rather than present a steady tone we should vary its intensity because the sudden increase of a tone is more stimulating to auditory sensitivity than a steady tone even though the latter may be very intense. A hard-of-hearing person who worked in an office next to a machine room told me that he heard the noise of the machines very prominently when he first went to work in the office but after a short time despite close attention to it, noted only a significant change or a sudden cessation.

Intensity of musical tones

Varying intensity

With this point in mind, in attempting to arouse auditory sensitivity, I would not present sustained single vowels initially, but would call them into the ear sharply, loudly and repeatedly. However, as I have noted previously, in cases with existing residual hearing a sustained speaking into the ear facilitates the correct hearing sensation.

Varying voice intensity

In the course of further training, in addition to speaking at varying distance from the ear, varying intensity of speech as expressed in loud, moderately loud and whispered speech is applied. In doing this, I practice alternating various levels of voice, always, however, in such a manner that the loud voice is still plainly audible to the listener at the greatest possible distance from the ear, the moderate level voice closer and the crisp whisper closest to the ear. In drilling with moderately loud speech and sharp whispering I make it a practice to reveal the phonemes, syllables or words to the subject in advance, and only in later drills would I use sounds or words without advance notice. If a

Varying distance from sound source

word at a given level and at a given distance from the ear is easily intelligible I gradually increase the distance from the ear repeating the word constantly. The more difficult phonemes become first indistinct and finally inaudible. The reverse procedure is employed in cases where a word is initially not heard or poorly heard; with decreasing distance from the ear the single sounds are perceived gradually according to the degree of their intelligibility. In car-

Various responses to speech sounds

rying out such exercises interesting observations can be made about the gradual transition from incorrect to uncertain and eventually to correct hearing; in one case / s / was heard as / d / at a distance of 70 cm., as / ds / at 60–20 cm., and only in the immediate vicinity of the ear as / s /; in similar fashion as the distance was increased this patient heard / s / as / ds / and eventually as / d /. Slowly increasing the distance between the speaker and the ear of the listener demonstrates the common phenomenon that auditory perception can be elicited from a greater distance than in the case where we gradually move from the range beyond the threshold of hearing into the hearing range. This phenomenon is even more pronounced in the perception of musical tones where the loss of perception of a tone can be different, depending on whether we move from the hearing range towards its limits or from beyond the limits into hearing range. For instance, a girl deaf to the highest tones could not hear f⁴, e⁴ to g³ when the highest tones were used first in the examination, whereas g³, a³, and $\overset{b}{h}$³ were perceived when the test began with a tone within the range of hearing, like c³, and there was a step-by-step progression of test tones toward g³.* I have made a similar observation, about which I shall report below, on a number of people concerning incorrect auditory response to specific tones near limits. Still in reference to the use in auditory training of loud, moderately loud and precisely whispered speech, it should be pointed out that the ease or difficulty of intelligibility of a word is not always reduced or enhanced in relation to the intensity of speech tones, but that quite noticeable variations may occur, particularly in the case of advanced auditory capability. Thus, sometimes a word spoken loudly is understood either not at all or indistinctly, while the same word spoken at a moderate level results in clear perception; and what is more, strikingly good hearing is manifested now and then with precisely whispered speech for those sounds and words which are not correctly perceived when moderate or loud speech is used. A man with acquired total deafness absolutely could not hear / e / and / I /, even after weeks of training. Then one day I presented both of these sounds first loudly then in a sharp whisper. He heard these sounds clearly for the first time since his illness when they were spoken quite close to the ear in a sharp whisper. From that time on, he could also recognize / e / and / I / with loud or moderate speech.**

Better hearing for weak stimuli

As I have mentioned previously, I recommend a hearing tube for auditory training only in exceptional situations

Use of a hearing tube

---

* See the same observation by *Knapp*, 48 Arch. f. Augen u. Ohrenhheilk, 1871, Bd. 2, Abth. 1.

** The striking fact that whispered speech can be significantly more intelligible than moderately loud speech I found to be specifically demonstrated in a luetic patient who was almost totally deaf to moderately spoken words but could perceive whispered speech well at a distance of 5 paces. (See *Arch. f. Ohrenhk.* 1880, XVI, p. 183.)

because it generally causes an all too powerful sound stimulus. At the very least, special caution is required which is generally not observed. Moreover, the ear trumpet alters the quality of the voice to a more or less considerable degree, so that the person instructed with the trumpet understands the naked voice poorly or not at all. Also, considering the reverse, the person who has been trained with the naked voice must first get used to an ear trumpet and will initially hear the voice with it more indistinctly than he did without it. Still, the ear trumpet may be useful in exceptional cases, for example, in self-instruction and here and there in order to compare one's own speech with that of a normal speaking person who in this case must likewise speak through an ear trumpet in order to achieve a similar quality of voice. More for scientific rather than practical tests, I sometimes used a three-part hearing tube in order to be able to feed a tone simultaneously to both ears and in this way to investigate the difference between monaural and binaural hearing.

Rate of Speech

Next to the intensity of speech, the rate of speech requires the greatest attention. At first the deaf mute is able to understand only sustained, distinctly articulated speech sounds. In the course of presentation of a word every single sound should be spoken into the ear in a sustained manner. The word Nase (nose), for example, is spoken as Nnnnaaaasssseeee in this case in such a way that every sound is sustained four times longer than in conventional speech. A common mistake when this kind of procedure in auditory training is carried out by a person not conversant with it occurs when only the first sound of a word or only certain sounds and not all sounds are given equal duration. Thus, the word Nase is given as Nnnase or Nnnnaaaase. In the course of this kind of stimulation, the sounds not given in sustained, carefully articulated fashion are considerably weaker and as a result, particularly at the beginning of such training, the hearing impression is not sufficiently clear. Plosives like / p / and / t / that cannot be sustained must be given with particular intensity.

As the drawn-out, distinctively articulated word is clearly understood then repetitions should be given with decreasing duration so that in this way the ear is gradually drilled in the understanding of conventionally paced speech. This is only attainable when hearing is already advanced and even then requires a good deal of painstaking instruction. Instead of single words, first short, then longer sentences are gradually introduced. The important practical value of such exercises is obvious and they should be instituted as soon as possible. With persons who acquired their deafness later in life, I frequently experienced just the opposite reaction in regard to understanding of slowly or rapidly spoken words. Sustained words or sentences were not understood at all or were heard with more difficulty than those more rapidly spoken.

More rapid speech

When I discuss the effect of systematic auditory training on those who acquired their deafness later in life, I shall return to a more detailed exposition of this phenomenon.

Effect of Pitch on Hearing Ability

In the implementation of auditory training, a fact very worthy of note is the occasional conspicuous manifestation of the dependence of auditory function on the pitch of the voice or musical tone. *Toynbee*[34] reports on a deaf mute girl who understood a high soprano voice best on her better hearing right ear and on her left ear was able to hear only a strong low-pitched voice. In one of my cases, I observed that a deaf girl could hear only a low-pitched voice and was totally deaf to a high voice.

The varying behavior in deafness for hearing of different tones was demonstrated by *Bezold*[35] in a detailed investigation:

Among the pupils of the Munich Institute for the Deaf, *Bezold* found 48 totally deaf ears: only 15 individuals were bilaterally totally deaf. In the remaining 108 partially deaf ears the deafness was either at one end or at both ends of the tonal scale, or also at various places and in various ranges within the tonal scale ("tonal gaps"). Anything from the smallest stretches of hearing up to the scale of 2½ octaves *Bezold* termed "island." As sound sources for the lower portion of the scale loaded tuning forks were used and for the upper portion 3 bird call whistles and the Galton whistle.

1. "Islands" were present in 28 sense organs; at times they appeared more rarely in the twice accented octave, but otherwise were present in all octaves.

2. There were "gaps" in the range from a half tone to 3½ octaves 20 times in all, 16 times singly and 4 times doubled.

3. In one instance there was deafness for the highest tones to g while the lower tones down to a lower octave were perceived.

4. In eight cases there was a simultaneous deficiency at the upper and lower tonal limits.

5. and 6. In 18 cases there were great deficiencies at the lower level of the tonal scale of 4½–7 octaves, in 33 cases from ½–4 octaves, while in both of these groups there were only negligible deficiencies present at the upper end.

In general, deficiencies were present more frequently and over a more extensive range at the lower part of the scale than at the upper end.

Elimination of partial deafness by auditory training

I have also frequently found in the deaf poor perception for single tones and especially for whole groups of tones. Yet, by concentrated practice with the appropriate tones I could, as a rule, improve perception of these tones and raise it gradually to that of the others. Hence, these drills furnish evidence that in such cases it is not a matter of a real loss of tone sensitivity but of an especially sluggish acoustic excitability which can be amenable to methodical practice. In these cases as in others a special intensity of the pertinent practice tone is often less essential than continuous prolonged stimulation. Thus, I have often found deaf mutes who could not hear a specific tuning fork or concertina tone even when presented strongly for a short time, but with sustained presentation of this tone for half a minute and sometimes for several minutes received an initially indistinct, hearing sensation which later became increasingly clearer. Once the tone has been clearly perceived, continued practice with it gives rise to an ever easier perception of that tone. *Magnus*[36] previously made a similar observation when in a case of acquired partial deafness he was able to eliminate the hearing loss by strengthening stimulation with the tones concerned through the use of resonators.

In many cases of deafness I have found concertina tones more suitable for stimulating the proper hearing sensation than tones produced by tuning forks since concertina tones can be presented in situations where a much greater intensity is required than tuning forks can achieve just as it is also easier with the concertina to produce the continuous sustained tones necessary to achieve more powerful stimulation for auditory sensitivity. I have repeatedly encountered cases where I have not been successful in eliciting an auditory response with a tuning fork, but have been able to do so with a strong concertina tone. Subsequently, it became possible to evoke the same response by the corresponding tuning fork tone, which initially had not effected a trace of hearing even with strong and sustained presentation. In addition to the stimulation of perception of a specific drill tone the tone can bring about perception of adjacent tones so that frequently 3–4 tones can be sufficient for excitation of tone sensitivity for an entire octave.

The use of specific tones results in a particular increase in hearing for these tones. Accordingly a deaf person understands a familiar voice better than a strange one, because there are, among other things, the variations in quality of the human voice. In fact, I have repeatedly come upon various individuals who could hear correctly sentences spoken by the instructor but yet could not do so with a strange voice particularly at first, and even appeared to be deaf to vowels. Based on this finding I always make an effort to include as soon as possible several people (men, women, children) in the instructional regime in order to accustom the deaf person to various voice qualities.

Importance of concertina tones

Simultaneous arousal of perception of several tones

Improvement of hearing for specific sound stimuli

Importance of using various voices

Partial Tone Deafness

Deafness involving single tones or a scale of tones can either occur within the tonal scale so that there are tonal gaps in auditory sensitivity, or it may be manifested by a narrowing of the normal frequency range of hearing.[37] In such cases there is a loss of sensitivity for the highest and lowest tones; the latter is called bass deafness and the former treble deafness. Generally tonal gaps extend over one tone or over several chromatically adjacent tones, however, several tonal gaps can occur isolated from one another. Thus in the case of *Magnus*, previously reported, the bass tones were heard well, there was a tonal gap from f^4 to $\overset{b}{h}^4$, within the twice accented octave 3 tones were not heard, followed by a series of well heard tones, and then again a loss of sensitivity for the highest tones.

Partial deafness has already been reported by older authors.* *Rosenthal*[38] mentioned a case where auditory sensitivity was limited to particular tones; *Wollaston*[39] observed a case of deafness extending over approximately 4 octaves; the same author knew about the frequent high-tone deafness, for example, for cricket chirps, also the fact that the limit of auditory perception is usually very sharply defined. *Itard*[40] reports partial deafness for particular classes of sound, namely a striking dissimilarity for hearing of noises, speech and music.

Helmholtz[41] reports a case of faulty perception for high tones and another for low tones. *Moos*[42] found a case of complete bass deafness that disappeared after eight days. *Schwartze*[43] noted a case of deafness for the highest tones that resulted from the blast of a locomotive whistle, similarly *Brunner*[44] in the case of somebody who had been hit with a stick in the region of the ear. *Knapp*[45] in one case established deafness in one ear for the piano tones g^3–g^4 after the onset of vertigo, vomiting and tinnitus, in a second case on one ear for the highest tones from b^3 and on the other ear from d^4 on; here the cut-off frequency for

---

* I have taken the following discussion of partial deafness from my article in *Schwartze's* "Handbuch der Ohrenheilkunde," I, p. 390

hearing was exceptionally variable; indeed, it seemed to lie higher when the tone frequency was gradually increased. However, it was more limited, that is, the hearing defect was considerably greater when the hearing test started with the high tones and then proceeded to the low tones. In a third case of *Knapp's* there was a loss of the highest and lowest tones, similarly in one of *Jacobson's* cases.[46] *Wolf*[47] found a deafness for f-sounds, among them, one after a shot and another after a kiss on the ear; besides these the same author reports on several cases of tonal deficit. *Burnett*[48] reports a case of deafness for all tones above C^3, *Gottstein*[48] above C^2, *Politzer* for the tones $\overset{b}{h}$ and f. There is currently under my observation an elderly music teacher who at age 20 from an unknown cause lost his perception for the highest tones of the piano to a^4; from then on within every two years perception for the next higher tone was lost so that the limit receded to a^3 within 15 years which tone was still heard in the year 1865; in 1868 there was a loss of hearing for g^3, in 1870 also for f sharp^3; in 1894 the limit was at a flat^2, and on some days at f^2. At times the limit of perception appears to be sharp so that the threshold tone struck weakly is clearly perceived while the adjacent tone presented very intensely is not perceived at all. The initial loss of perception manifests itself in a gradually increasing hearing impairment for the tone next in line to be affected so that now the tone is heard clearly and then again one-half tone too low. In one of my cases, a piano player frequently had a subjective auditory experience wherein a high tone g^3 or a^3 was especially affected. This tone, when struck on the piano appeared significantly muffled. After the subjective sensation had receded it would again be perceived as clearly as the other tones. Imperfect perception of a tone affected by subjective hearing sensation is also mentioned by *Hartmann*.[49]

We are familiar with the loss of the highest tones that accompanies aging as elderly people are frequently no longer aware of cricket chirp, similarly the high whistle of the bat, the high pitched *s*-tone (*Wolf*[50]), etc. More specific investigations concerning the loss of the highest and lowest tones with increasing age have been reported by *Zwaardemaker*.[51]

Albertoni[52] described the occurrence of an acoustic dalton-
ism namely where those with color blindness show an auditory defect. Two persons with color blindness for red
did not hear *g. Bonnafont,*[53] *Moos*[54] and *Lucae*[55] observed
frequent loss of the highest tones in cases of disease of the
sense organ; similarly for boilermakers (*Habermann*[56]).
Burckhardt-Merian[57] showed a diminished perception for
high tones with increasing pressure on the labyrinth, for
example, in cases of loading of the labyrinthine window,
as compared with elevation of threshold of sensitivity in
cases of loss of the ossicles.

The cause of partial tone deafness can be found in a
lesion of the auditory nerve or in the hearing center. With
reference to a partial lesion of the acoustic fibers, it might
be noted that although such a lesion is conceivable along
the path of the acoustic nerve trunk, observations to date
attribute this condition to an involvement of the peripheral
fibers and, indeed, adduce, according to the hypothesis of
Helmholtz disturbance of perception of the highest tones
to a lesion of the acoustic fibers in the basal turn of the
cochlea and of the lowest tones to a lesion in the apex.
Moos and *Steinbrügge*[58] found in a case of deafness for
high tones a carcinoma of the right anterior central con-
volution and atrophy of nerve fibers in the first turn of
the cochlea. *Baginsky*[59] states that a lesion in the base of the
cochlea results in a loss of perception for high tones while
a lesion in the apex has the same result for the low tones.
Corradi[60] had similar findings whereas *Stepanow*[61] could not
demonstrate any tonal deficit after destruction of the upper turn of the cochlea of the guinea pig. In a case of
boilermakers deafness, *Habermann*[62] found a thinning of
the acoustic nerve in the inner ear and a high degree of
change in the basal turn. This finding is in accordance with
Habermann's view that boilermakers can be severely hard-
of-hearing especially for high tones. As this author reasons
it is possible that atrophy of the related acoustic fibers
results from the particularly strong stimulation by high
tones associated with boilermaking. However, we also have
to take into account that lesions of the acoustic nerve in
general are frequently manifested first of all and most

severely in perception for the highest tones as is also shown in the pertinent findings for *Habermann's* ten cases.[63] On the other hand, a reverse relation can exist, namely profound deafness except for the highest tones.[64] In a case of deafness for the highest tones *Bezold*[65] found an atrophy of the nerves in the first turn of the cochlea and in another case where only one and one-half octaves in the middle of the tone scale were audible an atrophy of the first and second turn.

A partial deafness for tones, as has previously been noted, can also be due to a lesion of the acoustic centers in which a special significance attaches to the temporal lobe as has been shown in animal experiments and in pathologic studies. According to *Munk*[66] removal of the posterior portion of the temporal lobe close to the cerebellum effects a loss of the low tones while extirpation of the anterior portion of the temporal lobe close to the sylvian fossa causes a loss of perception for the high tones. See also the observations of *Moos* and *Steinbrügge*.[67]

In one case of transfer that I observed there was at first a crossover of perception for the highest tone from the hearing right ear to the otherwise profoundly deaf left ear; thereupon one tone after another disappeared in rapid succession from the right ear and emerged instead in the left ear, always adhering to the chromatic tone sequence.[68] With the crossover of the lowest tone the formerly hearing ear now appeared to be deaf while the previously deaf left ear had taken over the hearing capability of the right ear; 5–8 minutes later there was a return crossover of tone perception from the left to the right in exactly the same sequence as before. In this case the transfer was probably related to a change in the acoustic centers and not in the peripheral end organs. *Gradenigo*[69] describes two cases of deafness for middle tones which he attributes to an intracranial lesion. According to this author in cases of lesions of the acoustic nerve trunk perception for high tones is retained in the majority of cases but reduced in lesions of the labyrinth.[70]

Although every imperception to tone can be attributed to an auditory aberration every tonal deficiency or diminution of response to particular tones should not be interpreted as tonal deafness but can be due to a conductive obstruction of a mechanical kind. As I have gathered from relevant investigations specific tones can be especially attenuated in the course of their transmission while this may not be the case for the higher or lower tones adjacent to the affected tone. Hence, it appears that not all tones are equally affected by a conductive involvement. As we know, anomalies of the conductive system also affect the transmission of high and low tones in very different ways.[71] The experiments of *Burnett*[72] show that an increase in labyrinthine pressure above a certain intensity blocks the activity of the ossicles and the round window and that cessation of function occurs for high tones earlier than for low tones. *Lucae*[73] found that pressure on the round window membrane resulted in attenuation of transmission of the fundamental tone. *Siebenmann*[74] using the Valsalva procedure noted an upward shift of the frequency range and sharpened perception of the highest tones.

With increased tension of the tensor tympani the fundamental tone is generally attenuated. According to the observations of most authors,[75] this is accompanied by a sharpened perception of the high tones. In contrast, *Lucae*[76] notes increased perception of the low tones. In my investigations I have found that in the majority of cases at the moment of tensing of the tensor tympani there is a fading of perception for the highest tones and also to some extent of the lowest ones.[77]

Partial Tone Sensitivity

In contrast to partial tone deafness we need to mention partial tone sensitivity. In such cases, hearing function has ceased totally for all but a few single tones or sounds, or only very specific sound stimuli are still heard. In regard to the latter, a case of *Stahl*[78] and one of *Rosenthal*[79] are of interest, in the first case only the tone of a shawm was heard and in the other only that of a cow horn. *Gradenigo*[80] reports a case of deafness for tones of tuning forks while these same tones were heard even when produced less intensely by a trumpet or flute.

Lack of Musical Perception

A very noteworthy kind of auditory anomaly is the lack of musical perception. From childhood on many people appear to be incapable of discriminating among musical tones or they are unable to differentiate harmony from dissonance. This congenital dullness of the musical sense appears frequently in certain families and may be limited to one sex. Thus, *Earle*[81] knew of a family in which none of the male members could discriminate among musical tones. In other cases previous musical perception can be temporarily or permanently lost.

In this connection I cite a case of special interest. A very musically talented boy lost his fine musical perception in the course of a suppurative otitis of the middle ear in spite of only a moderate hearing loss for speech and watch tick. After the termination of the inflammation, hearing for speech appeared to be normal whereas there was no improvement in musical perception. Only a few months after the termination of the inflammation musical perception gradually returned and after a year attained its original level. *Nasse*[82] likewise observed an adverse effect of middle ear catarrh on musical perception. In a case I mentioned previously of gradual loss of perception for the high tones the affected tones lose only their tonal quality preserving, nevertheless, a certain musical sound effect which is the same for all tones but which allows an accurate differentiation from other sound stimuli, for example, where the sound from the impact of the hammer on strongly damped strings is recognized.

This kind of disturbance of musical perception may well be central in nature, and the hypothesis appears warranted that hearing for music takes place by way of specific pathways in the central nervous system the course of which is expounded in the noteworthy arguments of *Knoblauch*[83]. This opinion is supported by cases of sensory aphasia with preserved musical comprehension observed by *Wernicke*[84] and *Anton*[85]. In other cases disturbances of expressive ability in music occur simultaneously with the loss of speech, however, in observations till now, never by themselves. (*Frankl-Hochwart*[86])

Fluctuations in Hearing

Fluctuations in hearing occur regularly and show appreciable differences only in their intensity. They are contingent upon individual and various external circumstances. Thus, fluctuations in hearing occur frequently during the day either quite irregularly or associated with certain times of the day. Many individuals hear better before noon and others in the afternoon. Overall physical condition generally exerts a significant influence on hearing ability. Headaches especially are mostly associated with a significant aggravation of hearing, but hearing can also be considerably impaired as a consequence of various common illnesses without central symptoms. Of the external conditions that usually have an adverse effect on hearing, damp rainy weather above all, especially damp cold, should be mentioned. This can affect the hearing of the nerve-deafened in a similar way as with catarrhal ear conditions. Here I must emphasize particularly that this kind of diminution of hearing can also occur in such nerve-deafened individuals where no catarrhal complication of the middle ear is demonstrable. In several of my cases a significant decrease in hearing was manifested a few hours before a thunderstorm. A temporary increase or decrease of hearing without any perceptible cause occurs very frequently either for a short time or persisting for several days and even weeks.

Aggravation of hearing

The aggravation of hearing in such situations can be so significant that the achievements of weeks and months of auditory training seem totally lost. Such a persistent decrease in hearing can have an effect so depressing on pupil and teacher that, as I have repeatedly experienced, continued instruction was abandoned because of the presumed futility of attaining a lasting outcome. For this reason I want to call attention to the fact that, in all cases known to me till now, this kind of hearing loss, even after duration of several weeks, has proved to be temporary. In several cases where such periods of diminished hearing, even if almost complete loss of hearing occurred, I had to overcome it time and time again in one and the same individual.

I think it is advisable to call attention to such fluctuations in hearing right from the start and at the onset of such a period to pursue the training unswervingly, even to start all over again if the case requires it. These types of fluctuations of hearing occur in an especially striking way only with severe hearing impairment and appear less pronounced with improvement in hearing. They are nevertheless always evident even in developed hearing just as they can easily be recognized in non-nervous hearing impairment and even in a normal state of hearing.

In cases with initially existing slight hearing traces these can be totally lost during a state of auditory depression so that a hearing test administered at this time shows a total deafness which can also remain unaffected by auditory training and makes such a case appear to be hopeless, while hearing tests conducted at some other time may give evidence of traces of hearing and systematic training introduced at that stage can yield quite amazing results. Thus, there are two pupils in the Döbling School for the Deaf whom on the basis of my first hearing test I had to classify as totally deaf and who also remained unaffected throughout a prolonged period of continued auditory training. Renewed tests a year later showed a trace of hearing in both pupils which by continuous auditory training has now been improved to the point where they are actually able to hear words.

The hearing depression described here makes itself felt either for all sound stimuli and is therefore pervasive or it is only partial and is ostensibly confined to certain classes of sounds (speech, music, noise). There may also be within a particular class of sounds a lack of or reduced excitability by specific sound stimuli so that, for example, specific tones or speech sounds which were previously per-

Partial depression of hearing

ceptible were no longer heard or are perceived with particular difficulty while at the same time perception for other tones and sounds of speech remains unchanged. In a 23 year old individual I observed a peculiar case of a strictly partial deafness for the sounds of speech similar to partial tone deafness. In the course of auditory instruction she was able to hear the "r"-sound especially clearly; then, after a headache that lasted for several days, completely lost perception for "r" whereas the ability to hear the other speech sounds was unaffected. Only after many weeks of daily exercises with special attention to the "r"-sound did hearing for it gradually return and has remained unchanged after a year and a half.

Comparative hearing tests on both ears showed that fluctuations in hearing sometimes remain confined to one ear or are conspicuously more evident in one ear than in the other; at other times the fluctuations alternate between ears in such a way that with improvement in hearing in one ear there is a simultaneous aggravation of hearing in the other, and the developing hearing in the one ear coincides with diminution of hearing in the other ear. This type of alternation in hearing also occurs in middle ear involvements and sometimes appears, although to a very low degree, in normal sense organs as a physiological phenomenon.

Alternating fluctuations in hearing

In my experience I have quite frequently observed alternating fluctuations in hearing between ears in normal and pathological cases, as a matter of fact they can be considered as regular phenomena and concern hearing ability as well as subjective auditory sensations[87]. My observations indicate that subjective fluctuations of intensity of auditory sensations in both ears occur very frequently under normal conditions so that acoustic stimuli presented simultaneously to both equally sensitive ears are not always heard with the same loudness on both sides but appear louder sometimes to one ear then to the other or affect one exclusively[88]. Occasionally the diminution in the perceptual ability in one ear that occurs simultaneously with an increase in the other ear is gradual, and at other times these fluctuations appear quickly. While under normal conditions such fluctuations are generally rapid, in fact appear to oscillate, in pathological cases this kind of fluc- tuating auditory function can occur suddenly in both ears with great intensity and can remain permanent. Thus I have noted in several cases with symptoms of bilateral chronic middle ear catarrh where over the years hearing impair- ment developed significantly more in one ear than in the other that in the course of a few minutes or hours or in one case even in a moment a kind of permanent transfer suddenly took place. The previously poorer ear now heard better and the better ear appeared to sink to the level of the poorer ear. The change in hearing proved permanent for this patient who was in no way hysterical. I had a par- ticularly interesting case of this type, that of an 80 year old man who for 20 years was deaf to speech in his right ear and could understand words softly spoken into his left ear. Treatment did not result in any change of this condition. Then during one night without any known cause a transfer ensued; in the morning the patient showed deafness for speech in the left ear and comprehended softly spoken words in the previously deaf ear. This condition continued for four years until the patient died.

Unlike in the cases cited above, fluctuating hearing changes in both ears are, for the most part, only temporary, as was first observed by *Gelle*[89] in the so-called transfer case. A hysterical patient of mine whom I observed for a long time showed a complete anaesthesia on the left side of her body for all sensory stimuli. Among other things there was a total deafness in the left ear for all sound stimuli both by air and bone conduction; on the right ear she could hear a watch tick, normally perceived at a distance of 150 cm., at a distance of 36 cm; moderately spoken words were understood at a distance of 5 paces[90]. When a small horse- shoe magnet was placed on the insensitive left or right side of the head about five minutes later the patient reported a decrease in the subjective perception of a buzzing other- wise present in the sensitive right ear. Then there was an immediate diminution of perception in this ear for high tones and a gradual increase for these tones in the pre- viously insensitive left ear. Nevertheless, the left ear still

Transfer

remained totally insensitive to low tones; in a rapid inter-aural change perception for lower tones of the chromatic scale shifted from right to left until, with the shift of the lowest tone the right ear now appeared totally insensitive, while the left ear had taken over from the right ear the hearing for speech and watch ticks. Five to ten minutes later there occurred a transfer back from the left to the right ear precisely as before, first for the subjective sensation then for the high tones and finally for the low tones. The transfer recurred as a rule for a second and third time without further stimulation whereupon the previous condition returned, namely, that the left side of the patient showed insensitivity and hearing on the right side reverted to its pre-transfer state.

Physiological transfer

As I note in investigations of normal hearing similar transfer-like phenomena may occur physiologically[91]. When barely audible tones of a tuning fork are presented binaurally there is occasionally a subjective fluctuation of auditory sensation wherein a gradual increase in sensitivity occurs in one ear with simultaneous decrease in the other not equally for all tones but sometimes only for a few tones or a single tone. I have noted several instances where at a certain stage of the investigation physiological transfer corresponding to the chromatic tone scale was evident; namely, in the course of binaural tuning fork tests of those persons involved in the study one tone after another faded from one ear and for a few seconds or minutes were heard solely by the other ear. Then sensitivity for single tones returned to the first ear adhering to the chromatic tone scale sequence; then again with the same people there was an irregular "back and forth" fluctuation of hearing intensity for the various tuning fork tones or they were perceived equally strong by both ears. Similar manifestations are much more pronounced among the hearing impaired.

Transfer types among the hearing impaired

In 1875 I had occasion to observe a rather remarkable case of periodically alternating hearing[92]. A middle-aged man on the first day of examination showed a complete deafness in his right ear, in the left he could hear a pocket watch, normally perceived at a distance of 150 centimeters, at a distance of 20 centimeters. The next day the previously deaf right ear could hear the watch at 2 centimeters while at the same time a decrease of hearing in the left ear was evident. In the course of the following days there was a steady increase in hearing in the right ear and a decrease in the left so that on the eleventh day the left ear appeared to be totally deaf while the right ear approximated the previous hearing level of the left ear. From then on the hearing returned again to the left ear and the right ear gradually reverted to deafness. These alternations in hearing continued with a few interruptions for many years and were still manifest ten years after my first examination of this patient. The condition resisted every therapy. The patient did not want to undergo a recommended tenotomy of the tensor tympani.

Temporary fluctuations occur frequently in cases of diminished hearing in both ears, if not in the same pronounced and regular manner as for the case just cited. This is easy to demonstrate by comparative tests. With extended observation in such cases over a period of time we frequently find an entirely irregular pattern in the hearing ability of both ears in relation to each other, after which even for weeks, evidence of alternating hearing appears, namely, a periodic increase and decrease in hearing in one ear with a simultaneous change in hearing in the opposite direction in the other ear. Such regular fluctuations in hearing will again be replaced by irregular ones, and will again recur later, etc.

Acoustic fatigue and nervous symptoms

In the conduct of auditory training acoustic fatigue and other nervous manifestations demand our utmost attention. These nervous indications are expressed as anxiety, irritability, sleeplessness and very often in a dullness in the head that can precede a headache(s). At times the deaf person can pay diligent attention to his instruction for a short time and soon appear to be distracted or exhausted. At the same time, occasionally, however, as the sole symptom an acoustic fatigue occurs which can proceed from an increasing loss of previous hearing to the point of complete deafness, a condition similar to nervous asthenia. This phenomenon can fluctuate from time to time so that a particular phoneme or tone is sometimes heard or not heard, even with the most intense stimulation. However, this symptom is not always attributable to acoustic fatigue but can, as I have shown for normal and hearing impaired individuals[93], be due to fluctuations of intensity of auditory sensations.

The onset of acoustic fatigue is quite often signalled in the beginning as blurred, then incorrect hearing for the sounds of speech previously well understood followed by a gradual total loss of hearing.

The time course over which acoustic fatigue occurs varies among individuals. For some it can first be noted after a long lesson, for others, signs of fatigue are evident after the first few minutes. Occasionally only the initially presented phonemes or first syllables are heard correctly and already with the first repetition of these just distinctly heard speech sounds auditory uncertainty appears. In one case a deaf mute always heard an arbitrary concertina tone for a few seconds; whereupon hearing ability disappeared rapidly with continuing stimulation of that tone until only the stream of air was felt without any sensation of hearing. Frequently a short pause of one to several minutes is sufficient for complete recovery and sometimes longer pauses are required.

When particularly strong signs of acoustic fatigue or of various kinds of nervousness appear it is advisable to conduct the exercises for a short time only, say about 5 or 10 minutes, and not to undertake them too often during the day. Instruction may need to be interrupted completely for several days. Nevertheless, if possible, a longer break should be avoided because, as shall be discussed later, this will generally result in a decrease in the hearing that has been improved by auditory training.

Physiological acoustic fatigue

Acoustic fatigue can take place in normal as well as in pathological hearing. If, as *Dove*[94] has done, we present one of two equally tuned tuning forks of equal intensity steadily to the open ear canal of one ear and the other interruptedly to the other ear the hearing sensation on the latter ear is louder, an indication that the steady stimulation by the tone of the tuning fork causes an auditory fatigue of the first ear while a simultaneous interrupted acoustic stimulus in the second ear does not have this effect. *Müller*[95] noted that tonal sensation appears to be more hollow when a harmonic of the test tone is introduced into the ear before the test tone. My investigations have shown that in the case of equal hearing in both ears if the tone is presented till it fades in one ear and the tone is then presented to the other ear which up to that time had not been stimulated, it appears to be audible in that ear for several seconds[96]. However, in this situation the fatigue is confined only to the test tone so that an ear temporarily fatigued for a particular tone hears any other tone as clearly as the ear not exposed to tone stimulation before. Duration of fatigue in my normal-hearing subjects was generally only 2–5 seconds. In comparative tests of both ears I found that one ear can be fatigued sooner than the other and that in the case of asymmetrical hearing more rapid fatigue occasionally occurs in the better hearing ear. A more detailed investigation of these processes is possible by observing variations in the locus of the subjective "hearing field" in the head. I have termed that specific phenomenon "subjective hearing field" where simultaneous sound stimuli to both ears are very frequently heard neither in the right nor left ear but in the head. This "hearing field" is located in the middle of the head in the case of bilaterally equal or only marginally differing hearing in both ears. With varying intensity of tonal stimulation of both ears the sensation moves toward the more sensitive ear. Hence, the alteration of position of the hearing field allows the assessment of the relative behavior of auditory function of the right and left ear. *Eitelberg*[97] observed that there is more rapid fatigue in involvements of the acoustic nerve than in conductive cases.

Tactile perception

In the case of deaf mutes it is impossible at first to differentiate tactile from auditory perception by shouting

Differentiation from acoustic sensitivity

directly into the ear if only because frequently an auditory impression is generally unfamiliar to them and possible auditory sensations are often judged by the deaf person to be tactile. Nevertheless, it is possible when there are existing or potential traces of hearing to achieve an increasingly clearer recognition of the difference between an auditory and a tactile sensation. When this is done the auditory sensation is not readily recognized as such, but yet will stand out as a special sensation different from a tactile one. An attentive observer is frequently able to recognize the beginning of an auditory impression by noting a peculiar facial expression or a movement of the head of the deaf person. In cases of existing traces of hearing blowing strongly at the region of the ear without simultaneous articulation of the speech sound concerned results in an especially clear differentiation as opposed to the same sound shouted into the ear. In the same way in such cases discrimination takes place between the simple air stream of a concertina and the tone it produces. At the beginning of such a control experiment with the concertina a boy commented to me: "Now I feel only the air and then I detect the air and something else besides." The deaf person only learns in the course of subsequent training that this "something else" is an auditory sensation.

When hearing is unequal in both ears or if the traces of hearing are unilateral this kind of differentiation is especially evident to the deaf person; even in the presence of increasing acoustic fatigue the merely tactile impression appears rather conspicuously. Deaf persons who previously experienced definite auditory sensations know well how to differentiate them from tactile ones. When they speak individual sounds to themselves into a speaking tube deaf persons often notice that they hear them sometimes more, sometimes less clearly and sometimes not at all, in spite of the fact that the stream of air remains equally strong and that they know the sounds spoken.

Confusion of a tactile with an auditory sensation can be ruled out with certainty, if there is recognition of sounds in an ear from which the air stream has been diverted either by the speaking person holding his hand in front of his mouth or by inserting a partition between his mouth and the ear. Confusion of an auditory sensation with a tactile one can also be ruled out by increasing the distance of the talker from the ear. Furthermore, I should mention the frequently occurring cases where the ability to hear is frequency dependent, where, for instance, a sound spoken with equal intensity is sometimes heard and sometimes not heard depending on the pitch despite the equal airstream that impinges on the region of the ear in both tests.

In contrast it is worth considering a strange phenomenon here which, in my experience, can simulate hearing especially in training with various vowels. It involves a kind of sensitive localized feeling for specific tones and individual phonemes, particularly vowels, confined to specific places on the ear or head, so that depending on the tone or vowel directly presented to the ear a peculiar sensation appears located somewhere in the head that has nothing in common with an auditory sensation. As I have reported elsewhere, such a keen sensation sometimes accompanies the auditory sensation but occasionally appears alone, without it[98]. In the latter case discrimination among several vowels independent of any auditory sensation becomes possible. Certainly, it requires an acute talent for observation in the involved deaf person to note clearly how the localized sensations for the vowels differ, if his or her attention has not been alerted to that fact. In many cases it suffices simply to ask where the individual sound stimuli are sensed. Sometimes special drills are required for a more specific localization particularly when these points are very close to each other or even overlap, which makes their differentiation difficult. At other times localization is greatly facilitated and appears very pronounced when the sensitive loci are widely separated.

Sensitive localized perception of sound stimuli

Occasionally even with concentrated attention and repeated attempts, no separate loci of sensitivity are observable when various sound stimuli, for example, vowels spoken into the ear, always give rise to a sensation in the same location on the head or ear. In many cases only an auditory sensation is noticeable, while again in others, especially in cases of severe hearing impairment, only a sensory impression without a trace of auditory sensation is evident. In my observations till now this latter phenomenon occurs only in such cases in which a sensation of sound in response to a sound stimulus occurs when it is still below but very near to the threshold of conscious sound perception. In systematic investigations of arousal of hearing I noted that the gradual development of an auditory sensation can often be detected by the onset of certain specific sensation in the ear or especially in the head. Here the deaf person emphatically denies any auditory perception. Persons with deafness acquired later in life who had previously possessed clear auditory perception assured me that the acoustic stimuli concerned did not give rise to an auditory impression but to an unpleasant even painful sensation in the ear or especially in the head, mainly in the region of the forehead.

Thus it occurs often that acoustic exercises without any resulting auditory excitation produce a sort of dazed feeling in the head or even a headache, especially in the forehead. In cases of partial tone deafness I was able repeatedly to track this gradual diminution of auditory excitability more precisely. For example, in cases of deafness for the highest tones in the area of the frequency limit,

Sensitivity at frequency limit

slowly diminishing auditory excitability generally is evident in such a way that right at the frequency limit the appropriate auditory sensation is elicited only by strong and sustained stimulation by the border tone. Then, stimulated by tones lying beyond the limit, the subjects under study reported that during further tonal stimulation they did not hear anymore but experienced an unpleasant sensation in the head. It was more intense the closer the stimulating tone was to the tonal limit while tones lying further away in frequency were increasingly less likely to produce such a feeling so that with greater separation from the cut-off frequency even the most intense and painful audible tones did not produce any kind of identifiable feeling. If in reverse fashion we approach the frequency limit tone by tone the more distant tones do not produce any feeling while as the limit is approached gradually only a feeling but no auditory sensation is evident until the latter appears, either by itself or accompanied by sensitive impressions. In the case of a deafened girl who at times did not hear the highest tones at all or at other times perceived them weakly, strong and sustained b^3 stimulation on many days produced only a slight tone sensation, on other days resulted instead in headaches concentrated in the forehead; tones above c^4 usually could not produce any kind of feeling. With another almost totally deaf person the vowel / a / spoken loudly into the ear produced no kind of sensation whereas with / o / a strong tickling sensation in the ear was noted and from there radiated to the temporal region while simultaneously, but not always, a muffled kind of hearing for / o / was observed.

It is a generally known phenomenon that totally deafened persons at times experience a particular kind of painful sensation, not auditory in nature, for certain powerful tones or noises. In cases of this kind of effect of sound stimulation it is worth noting whether the sound stimulus is also close to the cut-off frequency.

There is substantial individual variation in the patterns of these sensitive loci, but it is for the most part consistent in the same person. The subjective loci are dependent on frequency and intensity. Sometimes they are distributed in different locations on the side of the head and at other times are layered at varying depths in one side of the head. Thus, low-pitched tones generally excite more in the region of the ear while, in contrast, higher tones frequently elicit a more medial sensitive feeling. These sensations, sensed more or less deeply, may make discrimination between a higher and lower tone by tactile means possible.*

Patterns of sensitive loci

In still other cases sensitive loci of perception for low tones lie more toward the area of the mastoid process and the high tones lie in the region of the entrance to the ear

---

* Also as I have observed with binaural stimulation "subjective fields" can appear in the middle of the head arranged in a kind of chromatic tonal scale, more specifically that normally the lowest tone has its localized subjective field in the occipital region and the highest tone in the region of the forehead. The subjective fields lying between them are always distributed in such a way that the higher tone is located in front of the lower. Even unmusical people with clearly discrete distribution of subjective fields were able to differentiate correctly the higher tone from the lower among various test tones, according to the distinctive arrangement of subjective fields. (Concerning subjective auditory regions *Pflüger's* Archiv. XXIV)

or sometimes on a plane that extends from the region of the temporal bone to the forehead where the loci for the high tones usually appear to be anterior to those for the low tones. In the case of a girl who formerly was totally deafened and who had improved with systematic auditory training speaking / a / into the ear generated a sensation that extended medially in a line from the entrance to the ear, with / I / the line deviated superiorly, with / e /, / u /, / o / it deviated inferiorly in steadily increasing steps. The pattern of these sensitive lines of sensation fanned out so that the uppermost line corresponded to / I /, the lowest to / o /, while / a / always maintained a horizontal direction. In another case / a /, / e /, / I / produced an inward extending line which terminated with / a / before / e / while / I / was experienced still deeper in the head; / o / was somewhat lower and / u / extended further downward than / o /.

Their displacement and dependence on tonal intensity

In some cases there are displacements in the loci and in the directional course of these sensitive points; for example, in the case just mentioned, on some days / o / was sensed uppermost, / a / in a horizontal line, / I / somewhat lower, / e / below / I /, followed by / u /. In another case deviations existed only for / e / in the course of the sensitive lines; / a / always penetrated from the ear towards the back of the head, / e / sometimes directly deeply into the depth of the ear, on other test days, inward and somewhat to the back, / I / always towards the back of the head, / o / produced "a reverberation in the whole ear," / u / penetrated the ear similarly to / e / although not as deeply.

With regard to the dependence of the sensitive points on tonal intensity a weaker tone usually generates a smaller subjective field than does a stronger one. In this situation the various tones overlap in a pattern of corresponding circular areas but their foci are, nevertheless, more or less discriminable. Sometimes varying intensities of a specific tone can induce lateral displacement of the sensitive perceptual field. Thus, in one case the sensitive field for one and the same tone presented weakly to the ear was localized in the temporal region but with more intense stimulation was sensed in the region of the forehead where with especially strong stimulation a kind of reverberant sensation appeared; when, in this case, a specific concertina tone was presented, first weakly then gradually increased in strength, the sensitive field that at first was concentrated over the ear gradually moved anteriorly to the forehead. In the same case the sensitive points for the different tones were localized at various depths, specifically the lowest tones outward and the highest tones inward toward the middle of the head. In another case as sound intensity was increased the sensitive field for / a / moved from deep in the ear towards the occiput and similarly for / e /, yet for / a / a spherical extension of the field was observed while for / e / only a perceptional line was noted; / o / penetrated the ear less deeply with weak than with stronger stimulation, for / I / the field always was concentrated at the entrance to the ear, regardless of the strength of stimulation and / u / did not stimulate a localizable sensitive point. The following observation may serve as a further illustration: Louder stimulation moves / a / from the ear towards the occiput, softer stimulation directly in the ear causes the sensitive field to "come apart;" / e / behaves like / a /, only for / e / there is no sensitive area but a sensitive line, / o / penetrates directly into the ear although with soft stimulation less deeply than with loud speaking into the ear; for / I / the sensitive point is localized more outward than for / o /; / u / generates a diffuse indeterminable sensitive field.

Aside from the intensity of the sound stimulation the strength of the sound sensation can influence the subjective sensitive points. With stimulation by constant intensity but with unstable sensing capability changes in loci are observed.

When a word spoken into the ear is clearly heard many subjects report a subjective sensitive field in the temporal or frontal region whereas with distorted hearing the field is not precisely localizable. Especially worthy of note in this connection is the report of a keenly observant severely hearing-impaired girl who underwent systematic auditory training for months. One day when I spoke the word "Clavier" (piano) at a distance the girl thought she heard "Lampe" (lamp) but in so doing stated that the subjective field was not localized in the frontal region as usual but in the temporal area. When I called the word "Lampe" there was a clear sensitive field in the frontal area. After repeated

Locus of the sensitive area in clear and distorted hearing

presentation of the word "Clavier" she understood this word also quite clearly and the sensitive field was observed likewise in the frontal region. Another time "Polster" (cushion) was heard as "Sonne" (sun) with only / o / clearly perceived in the ear without an indication of any sensation in the frontal area which the patient termed "quite strange;" with repeated presentation of the word "Polster" a gradually increasing perceptional field in the frontal region emerged, until finally the word "Polster" was correctly understood and simultaneously the perceptual field which the girl had regularly observed in conjunction with clear hearing, became distinctly prominent.

The nature of the effect
of systematic auditory training on hearing

I now turn to a discussion of the nature of the effect on the sense of hearing that can be attributed to systematic auditory training. In this connection we consider (1) Excitation and further development of auditory sensations and (2) Developing interpretation of achieved auditory perceptions by gradual separation of various sound stimuli and by learning the meaning of verbal stimuli. Although the expression "totally deaf" is employed in referring to many deaf mutes and although many pupils in schools for the deaf are so labeled, nevertheless, an actual complete deafness even among deaf mutes is rare because usually there is evidence of residual hearing, at least in one ear. Thus, I have come upon only 3 cases of total deafness among 100 pupils of the Vienna School for the Deaf in Döbling. They could not perceive vowels, tuning fork or concertina tones or noises. Yet, even in these cases, only after repeated and lengthy sustained sound stimuli would it be possible to judge whether there is indeed a complete loss of auditory sensation or if the sense of hearing is just hard to excite. In the interest of the deaf person, the importance of this latter condition cannot be emphasized enough and the more experience I have gained in this connection the less often do I encounter a case of "total deafness" that cannot be influenced.

Excitation and further development of auditory sensation

The efforts to excite the first traces of hearing in an apparently totally deaf individual are fraught with the greatest difficulty. They require complete dedication to the task and, above all, inexhaustible patience. But the greater the energy devoted to it the greater is the satisfaction with the final success which fortunately occurs more frequently than one would initially expect. When we keep in mind that with the sign of the first traces of hearing the groundwork is laid for further development of the auditory sense, we become aware of the great responsibility we take on when we terminate systematic auditory training prematurely in cases where perhaps with more perseverance, success would have been possible. Hence, I have tried especially to demonstrate the potential for a result even with the supposedly totally deaf who were, as a rule, excluded from any attempt to develop their hearing ability because any such endeavor was considered to be hopeless. In fact, surprisingly good results are possible even in these cases which I have observed not only in my subjects but also in a considerable number of the deaf at the Lower Austrian State School for the Deaf in Döbling (Vienna) under the direction of *Lehfeld*, the first institution to undertake systematic auditory training for the apparently totally deaf based on the principles presented here.

Importance of first indication of hearing

Auditory development resulting from systematic auditory training usually progresses more rapidly in cases of already existing residual hearing, especially where there is partial or complete hearing for vowels, than in cases where there is very slight hearing to begin with. Even more favorable are those cases in which there is already hearing for words where after some exercises there is comparatively rapid progress to hearing for sentences, an observation quite familiar to experienced teachers of the deaf.

All-around development of the sense of hearing

Development of the auditory sense associated with systematic auditory training is frequently not confined to that sound source that has been employed in the training but extends over the whole range of hearing. Thus, with training concentrated exclusively on speech, hearing is improved not only for speech but along with it there is a gradual increase of perception for sounds not previously perceived such as for tuning forks, bells, and various musical tones for which there was no specific emphasis in the training. The following cases illustrate this: A 17-year-old congenitally deaf boy who after several months of training with speech sounds demonstrated partial understanding of sentences suddenly became aware one day of the previously unfamiliar low tones emitted by the bells of a nearby church. Other deaf persons, in the course of speech training heard the tones of a barrel organ, electric signal bells, a locomotive whistle, etc. A 23-year-old congenitally deaf girl who after 6 months' training with speech was able to hear several short sentences, experienced for the first time in church a strange sound sensation which moved her so powerfully that she began to cry. As it turned out, it was the sound of the organ which up to that time she had never heard.

At other times increasing clearer perception of noises of the street, in buildings where there are machines, etc. is gradually facilitated by training that employs speech exclusively. A 32-year-old man[99] who had acquired total deafness at a mature age and who had experienced a significant improvement in hearing through auditory training reported to me that especially after dark when he lacks visual control he thinks he hears a rapidly moving carriage in the immediate vicinity, while it later turns out that the carriage is still many meters away. Before his instruction this man did not hear the rumble of a carriage at all and was often in danger of being run over.

Just as our experience shows that training employing speech exclusively carries over to musical tones the reverse also takes place. The procedure described earlier employs musical tones, especially of the concertina, for the stimulation of hearing for speech.

Auditory function developed through acoustic training concentrated on one ear can carry over to the other ear not so trained. I have observed several cases in which with exclusive training of one ear gradually increasing traces of hearing appeared in the other which eventually developed into a more or less distinct hearing for vowels. This kind of transfer effect on the contralateral ear varies in individuals and occurs in many cases only in the later stages of instruction occasionally not until hearing ability in the target ear is already well advanced. A deaf person with an apparent total deafness in the left ear who after a few training sessions clearly discriminated the vowels / a / and / I / exhibited the following: with auditory training concentrated only on the right ear there was considerable development of hearing; in the left ear which I used as a control only occasionally there appeared to be no trace of hearing. In the course of continued training of the right ear gradually increasing traces of hearing in the left ear were manifest until finally the left could discriminate clearly / a / from / I / without special drills. In another case a specific musical tone was heard in the left ear only after it had been directed for some time to the right ear immediately before. On the other hand, I have observed several cases in which no such transfer of training could be demonstrated.

Concerning the effect on the sense of hearing of one side resulting from a reduction or an enhancement of the auditory function in the other ear

The effect which the weakening and diminution of hearing in onè ear can have on the auditory function of the other has already been suggested by *James Sims* who observed a reduction in hearing in one ear caused by obstruction of the other ear[100]. *Eitelberg*[101] in 12 cases of accumulation of cerumen in one ear tested the hearing in the other before and after evacuation of the cerumen. The investigation indicated that after evacuation the hearing for watch ticks in the untreated ears increased in 8 cases from 2 to 104 cm., in one case diminished by 43 cm. and

Training the other ear

in 3 cases remained unchanged; however, in 2 of the latter 3 cases, evacuation resulted in a quite negligible or no improvement in the treated ear itself. In general, elimination of hearing impairment in one ear enhanced auditory function in the other.

Concerning the effect that excitation of one ear can have on the auditory function of the other I have reported elsewhere that unilaterally practiced training on one ear can carry over to excitation of the other ear excluded from stimulation[102]. Quite similar observations can be made on the eye. *Volkmann*[103] has reported evidence that improved ability to sense the location of a specific point on the skin achieved by training results in an improvement of local sensing of the corresponding point on the other side of the body that has not been involved in the training. Furthermore, *Weber*[104] found that muscle training for one side of the body proves to be beneficial for the corresponding muscles on the other side. Concerning the influence that auditory training concentrated on one ear can have on the other ear *Eitelberg's*[105] thorough studies found that out of 18 cases, 12 experienced a gradually increasing, usually temporary improvement in hearing in the ear not directly involved, 3 cases showed no change in auditory function and 3 cases even a diminution of hearing for a short time.

Groundwork for auditory comprehension

Beyond excitation and further development of auditory sensations systematic auditory training makes a gradual distinction of the impressions of hearing possible, and leads to their increasingly correct interpretation.

Initiation of interpretation of achieved auditory perceptions.

Tests of hearing for musical tones, for example with the concertina, indicate some residual hearing in a comparatively significant number of the deaf, indeed, even occasionally surprisingly good hearing. Although these individuals are able to detect the presence of speech sounds, they are not able to discriminate among them and are thus incorrectly judged to be deaf. Already in my early tests it struck me that subjects apparently deaf to speech sometimes exhibited a special sensitivity to sound stimuli and even exhibited a painful sensation or fright when a louder sound was presented. Every teacher of the deaf knows cases in which deaf children correctly identify familiar phonemes or several words even at a distance but otherwise appear to be deaf to speech. How large is the number of deaf mutes who always receive hearing impression by the various vowels or syllables spoken but do not understand them! I point out an illustrative instance out of many such observations: A very intelligent 23 year old lady who, through the efforts of the late Privy Councillor *Renz* had enjoyed conscientious deaf-mute instruction and who was presented to me as apparently totally deaf (from birth) told me that when vowels were spoken into her ear she always had the same auditory impression, that of a muffled sounding / E: /. I then selected the vowels / a / and / I /, each time before speaking into her ear indicating to her which of the two vowels I was going to say. In the course of a few minutes she was able to discriminate between / a / and / I / and in a few days following the same procedure all of the vowels were correctly discriminated by both ears. Within the short span of a few weeks other deaf persons were able to hear and to repeat correctly a series of words.

Similar phenomena can be observed related to varying hearing for diverse musical tones. As I have observed repeatedly, tones lying far apart on the tone scale may be heard but not be perceived as distinctive tones. However, after a short time of training, sometimes only after extended training, a continual improvement in auditory discrimination occurs to such a degree that now tones close together on the tonal scale can be recognized as being different where originally even tones several octaves apart could not be differentiated. In one case two tones that were two octaves apart could not be identified as distinctive tones, while already a few days later with continuous training, tones one octave apart and after a few weeks even tones a musical third apart could be discriminated.

Discrimination of tones

It is certainly clear that quick hearing results of this kind cannot be ascribed to a sudden development of the sense of hearing but rather to a proper interpretation and

Psychic deafness

differentiation of auditory impressions already attained. Here the hearing ability as such is not involved but primarily the increasing understanding of auditory discrimination.

Krügelstein[106] notes that children who live on isolated farms and homes in the first four years of life often appear to be totally deaf mute; this supposedly occurs namely in mills where the constant noise can dull the sense of hearing even in otherwise normal people. *Krügelstein* found congenital retardation and lack of practice in hearing and speech but no organic defect as the cause of the presumed deafness which later, as a consequence of instruction in school, can be eliminated. *Deleau* argues that a deaf mute, if he could hear speech for the first time, would not be able to understand the spoken words just like someone hearing a foreign language for the first time[107]. *Bonnafont* mentions that persons who suddenly hear better find it difficult to discriminate among sound stimuli and must at first be taught to discriminate[108]. In one case 4 weeks of training were necessary. This is comparable to the case of a girl who was operated on for bilateral cataracts by Dupuyfren (1829) and who afterwards required a month to differentiate among visual stimuli.

Benedikt mentions cases in which "the acoustic pathway from the periphery to the center for perception of non-speech sounds and the center itself can be more or less intact while transmission or the center for perception of articulated stimuli and, perhaps, even for musical concepts can be defective."[109] *Benedikt* maintains and correctly so, that many people are judged to be deaf or severely hard-of-hearing because they show a congenital or acquired inability to perceive speech while their perception for simple noises and non-speech sounds is obviously normal. Since in such cases the illness involves only a particular portion of the central ramification of the acoustic nerve he considers training as the only possible treatment.

Benedikt notes a second possibility that sometimes after a long standing acquired hearing impairment speech is lost and what is more, even where the pathology is peripheral, the ability to perceive speech disappears. "If after years, e.g. as a consequence of therapy, there is a significant improvement and if the pathology was especially peripheral the capability to hear noises and single sounds is improved or established. If in such cases speech perception is not improved at all we cannot say that the physical basis for speech perception has not improved just as we cannot deduce that someone who does not understand Chinese is hard of hearing!" "We must view similarly those patients who show a normal or slightly decreased sensitivity to noise but who have not had their capability for perception of articulated speech restored. These patients can hear articulated sounds the combinations of which constitute spoken language but they cannot understand because they have never learned or have forgotten the association of articulated sounds with certain images and concepts. We can restore to them the ability to comprehend language aurally only by training of the kind that occurs naturally in children, that is to speak and to elaborate words as frequently as possible and to teach them somehow that these words are associated with specific concepts." In his textbook on electrotherapy *Benedikt* refers to an instructive case of this kind and reports on two additional cases where speech training achieved good results.

I have reported the statements of *Benedikt* concerning this auditory disability in detail because they are basic to the current assessment of this problem and serve to illuminate clearly the nature of this condition. For a more thorough study of this disorder we are indebted to *Heller*, Director of the Institute for the Blind on the "Hohe Warte" in Vienna[110]. *Heller* terms the inability to associate a perceived word sound pattern with the related concept as psychic deafness with physical hearing. According to *Heller* children with this kind of disorder can be recognized by such behavior as reacting to music, developing a private language and sometimes by demonstrating significant residual speech, e.g. ability to pronounce individual syllables—none of which occurs in genuine deafness. In agreement with *Heller*, among others, I am convinced that proper pedagogical training can achieve surprisingly favorable results often in a relatively short time. An incorrect assessment of this acoustic disorder that results in the kind of instruction suitable for deaf mutes can lead to an incalculable impairment of auditory function because with the lack of auditory stimulation children who are originally only psychically deaf will be trained to be physically deaf or deaf mutes.

Mixture of physical and psychic deafness

More frequent than the cases of pure psychic deafness described above are mixtures of physical and psychic deafness. Virtually every child who has some remnants of or partial hearing and who has received no acoustic stimulation and attention is deficient in understanding his auditory sensations. With systematic auditory training the groundwork for development of hearing goes hand in hand with the development of auditory comprehension so that in the gradual expansion of auditory range, physical and psychic hearing are affected together. A careful test of the hearing status of deaf mutes does, however, reveal a situation worth noting in which among deaf mute children such children are often found who do not belong in a school for the deaf but who require special psychic auditory training. Segregation of these from the true deaf mutes is an urgent humanitarian imperative.*

Association of concepts with acoustic impressions

I have come across several very noteworthy phenomena in particular cases concerning the pattern and manner of developing interpretation of stored acoustic impressions. What is primarily an inability to associate a correctly heard and repeated word with its appropriate meaning emerges especially with intelligent and otherwise educated deaf mutes. A mentally very alert deaf mute girl after some acoustic lessons repeated the word "Anna," her sister's name, correctly after it was said into her ear but did not associate the word with her sister. She performed similarly when other words were used, that is, failed to associate well perceived words with their related concepts. It was very interesting to observe her surprise when I made clear to her to whom "Anna" actually referred. One could see that from

---

* From the year 1896 on, all such cases in Lower Austria will probably be placed in an institution for the feeble minded established by the Lower Austrian Diet, and form a separate department where such cases will be trained and instructed by methods suited to them.

that moment on a new mental domain had been opened to the child. From that time on the girl strived steadily and with increasing success to associate a word heard with its related concept. In other cases, however, words heard for the first time were associated with concepts spontaneously, or a changeable pattern was evident so that the meaning of single words was sometimes understood and at other times not understood.

The emergence of auditory images was addressed previously. We pointed out how through acoustic training for particular words and sentences auditory patterns can be acquired which become increasingly clearer with continued training and can be differentiated one from the other, while at the same time those not drilled remain unintelligible. In a quite similar way melodies can be "imprinted" where the subject otherwise can hear only isolated tones but not their harmonic patterns. A patient whose deafness was acquired late in life could perceive only isolated tones from an orchestra or from military music and got nothing when a familiar folk song was played to her on the zither. With repeated playing in parts and finally after the song was played to her 20 times in uninterrupted sequence she heard it clearly. From then on this woman was able to hear and recognize this song also when played by an orchestra without knowing beforehand when it was going to be performed. On the other hand she could hear only isolated tones of other orchestral pieces and only after several months of auditory training was she able to hear melodies and finally entire pieces.

Very interesting observations are possible concerning the psycho-physiologic process involved in the triggering of an auditory impression in cases of the deaf or almost completely deafened. Very frequently the understanding by a deaf person of a word that is already familiar as a result of previous training is conspicuously delayed so that it takes a few seconds or still longer for a word to be comprehended. A deaf girl told me that she had the impression that the acoustic trigger seemed to be centered in the region of the temporal bone. Several individuals in whom the onset of auditory awareness was greatly delayed had

Emerging auditory patterns

the impression that they were not dealing with an actual auditory registration but that they gradually or suddenly became conscious of the word. Some such cases must apparently first recollect the phonemes or words. I got the impression of a person who has not heard a word or sentence but to whom the words in question come to mind. I picked up this phenomenon most strikingly in the case of a severely hearing-impaired individual who could not understand a question after many repetitions but to whom after about fifteen minutes the question "suddenly came to mind".

In all such cases it must be determined specifically whether there really is a delayed onset of auditory perception or whether the individual just combines single phonemes or syllables heard into words and sentences, a process that sometimes requires a long time. I have been assured by several very intelligent deaf persons that the frequently used strategy of combination and part guessing of spoken words does not apply in this case. The verbal signals are first not heard at all and only gradually do they come to be perceived. "It seems to me that I hear nothing by ear and then all of a sudden I know what was said," a girl almost totally deaf to speech commented. A 32-year-old deafened man who lost his hearing at 28 and who had improved significantly with auditory training told me that frequently he did not understand a word or sentence but with intensive concentration what had been spoken sometimes "occured to him." As far as I have observed, this phenomenon of delayed recall appears most significantly at the beginning of an awakening of hearing and normally does not occur that conspicuously with increased auditory capability but can be often demonstrated with some close attention. It is a common observation in general even in the case of normally hearing people who listen intently that isolated words and sentences belatedly fall into place. By the way, similar phenomena occur in visual perception. It has often happened to me that I did not recognize an otherwise familiar object at first glance but only after several seconds and sometimes even later do I realize with certainty what the fleeting object was. Being myopic, I often have the opportunity of observing that the same occurs in cases of blurred vision. Of course, inferring may play a significant role in this situation so that in the case of belated recognition of fleeting or unclearly seen objects cognition sometimes plays the major role.

In the cases where the auditory impression necessary to achieve understanding of a word or sentence spoken into the ear was insufficient I was interested in gathering more specific data concerning the auditory process involved. In this regard, the following was reported to me: A clearly understood word is apparently heard deep in the ear while syllables and words that are not understood give rise to a confused auditory sensation wherein singly heard phonemes seem to whirl around among themselves and do not connect into syllables. At times this phenomenon abates, the isolated phonemes blend into syllables and the spoken word is slowly understood. A severely hard-of-hearing person told me that in listening to a sentence he did not hear clearly, he experienced a sensation as if single words fanned out in radial fashion from the speaker and only that syllable was understood that was in the direction of that radius which extended from the mouth of the talker to his ear. "It seems to me," he said "that I would hear different words if I stood elsewhere."

When speech is presented at some distance from the ear hard-of-hearing people frequently have the impression that the sound passes by the ear without penetrating it as though it came from a long distance. In the case of partial hearing only individual phonemes of a word or individual words of a sentence apparently enter the ear and are perceived there while poorly perceived or imperceptible phonemes penetrate only superficially or not at all. Thus a severely hard-of-hearing girl sensed the / e / of the word *Fenster* (window) deep in the ear, the / s / and / r / likewise in the ear but also somewhat in the region of the forehead while the remaining, unheard phonemes appeared to yield an undefinable hearing sensation at the entrance to the external auditory meatus which penetrated no further into the ear. With repeated presentations of a word or sentence a gradually increasing auditory perception is often realized in a way that more and more phonemes are aurally perceived within the ear until finally the right verbal construction is recognized.

I now turn to answer several questions of practical importance about systematic auditory training which suggest themselves almost automatically to everyone involved in the subject, namely: For which cases is such training suitable? How long should it be undertaken? What is its practical value and expected outcome?

Suitability for auditory training

First of all I address the question: For which cases is systematic auditory training suitable? The answer to this question has the most immediate significance for the deaf, in fact, can possibly be decisive for the course of their entire life. In this context there is the great danger that if we take only theoretical considerations into account and are indifferent to practical experience, a large number of the deaf will be considered inaccessible to an acoustic education right from the beginning. That such a fear is not unfounded I can plainly deduce from some remarks by Professor *Politzer* about the value of systematic auditory training as recommended by me. *Politzer* said at the XI Medical Congress in Rome (1894) "that before we consider the possibility of improvement of residual auditory capability we should look at the pathological-anatomical changes in the ear of the deaf person. Involved here for the most part are terminal processes (obliteration, ossification, atrophy, etc.) which all positively cause deafness the improvement of which we can only consider if improvement could be achieved in the anatomical conditions. This is unthinkable in the case of irreversible processes. Improvements reported by a number of authors lack any anatomical explanation."[111]! At the scientific congress in Vienna (1894) *Politzer* expressed similar sentiments and indicated that a large number of the deaf with radical changes in the hearing mechanism (about 70 percent (!)) should absolutely be excluded [112].

Theoretical considerations

I must reject most emphatically such a purely theoretically based opinion. Supported by my continually increasing practical experience I can assert that the outcome of systematic auditory training is initially unpredictable. In all cases the attempt should be made and no deaf person should be excluded automatically from instruction on a trial basis. Even a case that at the outset appears quite hopeless can with patience and perseverance in systematic auditory training manifest a development of hearing that sometimes increases to a surprising degree. We certainly cannot specify in individual cases of congenital or acquired deafness in what manner or to what extent the auditory nerve or centers are affected; even in the case of a destructive process of the sense organ it is at present hardly ascertainable whether only a part or perhaps all of the sound processing mechanism is involved. But even if only a part of the sound processing organ and its associated pathways have been preserved there is the possibility for systematic training of the residuum to stimulate auditory function to an extent that is, of course, quite undeterminable in advance. Furthermore, there is the possibility that processes involving the acoustic nerve and centers do not destroy these, but only impair or suspend their function, and that this function can be restored by training employing auditory gymnastics. In every individual case we have to be mindful of our total uncertainty about the condition of the acoustic center and have therefore to determine, everytime by means of trial therapy whether and to what extent auditory function can still be restored. This conclusion might be logically drawn from the following comment by *Politzer*: "Despite a good many histologic findings the pathologic anatomy of deafness is still very incomplete. Especially still little known are the changes in the central pathway of the acoustic nerve that cause deafness."[113]

Practical experience

Of particular value in this connection are the most recent reports of *Mygind* because they are supported by a number of his own valuable investigations[114]. *Mygind's* compilation of pathological findings indicates most clearly our still incomplete knowledge of the pathology of deafness, a point *Mygind* stresses especially. How can it be possible at

Histologic findings in deafness

Results of auditory training for deafness due to meningitis and other diseases

this time to have a clear picture of the pathologic processes in the auditory organs and in the central acoustic region when according to Mygind's compilation, up to the year 1893, only 150 pathological findings are available to us, a great part of which is very incomplete, especially with regard to the acoustic nerve and centers.

Consequently the effect of auditory training on the sense of hearing can be determined in each individual case only by experience. Training on a trial basis is therefore indicated in every case of congenital or acquired deafness. Putting this into practice I have attained hearing results among cases of acquired deafness, mostly in cases of deafness following cerebrospinal meningitis, scarlet fever, typhus, trauma and in two cases of deafness following shock.*

Especially remarkable to me are the results with those deafened by cerebrospinal meningitis since this disease accounts for a large contingent of deafened children put in schools for the deaf. Until now it has been assumed that the prognosis in these cases is unfavorable especially when deafness persists for months after termination of the meningitis. Certainly the uselessness of auditory training is indicated in cases deafened by cerebrospinal meningitis where the acoustic nerve and the acoustic centers have been completely destroyed. This has been demonstrated by histological findings. However, in my experience till now a majority of cases appear to be more or less responsive to acoustic management. As a matter of fact I achieved some of my best hearing results in several such cases among which there were some whose deafness had persisted unchanged for many years.

Among some persons deafened by scarlet fever and diphtheria acoustic exercises turned out to be ineffectual. In these cases there was probably a complete destruction of the auditory nerve as can happen, for example, when diphtheria invades the labyrinth. In other cases of deafness following diphtheria and scarlet fever I have been able to influence the sense of hearing favorably.

---

* In one of the two cases the deafness had existed for 22 years; it involved a man of 24 who was put on a glowing hot pot when he was two years old and was deaf from that moment on.

As has been mentioned previously, systematic auditory training can also improve hearing in those cases in which deafness has been present for many years. I have achieved hearing results through systematic auditory training in individuals 20–30 years old with congenital deafness or deafness acquired in earliest childhood.

To be sure it should be assumed that arousal of the sense of hearing is more difficult after long years of inactivity than in cases of shorter duration. Because of this, training should be begun as soon as possible. With deaf mutes in the first five or six years of life as well as with retarded deaf mutes where formal systematic instruction is not feasible we should at least try frequently during the day to introduce into their ears all kinds of sounds especially musical tones. *Wolff* recommends that with the beginning of instruction in speech, spelling, language and reading auditory training should be introduced simultaneously. Since September, 1894 this integrated method of instruction has been practiced with very satisfactory results at the Döbling School for the Deaf.* The advantages of this method lie on the one hand, in the possibility that the acoustic stimulation will contribute to auditory excitation and, on the other hand in the assistance given by the ear to phonetic instruction which is always dependent on the current state of hearing. This is an important fact from the practical viewpoint that I shall later consider in more detail.

Length of auditory training

I now turn to answering the second question: For how long should systematic auditory training be carried on?

The need for special auditory training grows out of the difficulty in exciting auditory sensations. As long as common sounds of the environment do not cause auditory sensation to cross the threshold to auditory perception spe-

---

* *Kühnel*, Teacher of the Deaf, who undertook this instruction in the academic year 1894/95 used a mirror which enables the child simultaneously to observe lip movements while speech is presented to the ear.

cial acoustic stimulation must be employed until finally in the individual case the sense of hearing is developed to a stage where common sounds are perceptible.

Stimulation of auditory capacity

The normal ear constantly receives auditory impulses generated by various sound stimuli and is never completely dormant. But depending on the degree of his hearing loss the hard-of-hearing person finds himself in a more or less silent space in which little or no sound reaches him. As a result, for the imperfectly functioning sense organ the lethargy induced by inactivity becomes more aggravated. If this sluggish condition is successfully attacked by systematic acoustic stimulation and perceptual ability increases it is obvious that the improved functional capability can be maintained and further improved only by continued auditory stimulation, whereas if it is dropped there will probably be a relapse into the previous dormant condition. Accordingly our experience shows that deaf mutes who have attained a significant improvement through auditory training often revert rapidly to their previous state of deafness when auditory training is discontinued especially in the beginning of the regime. This is the case as long as the degree of such development of the auditory sense has not reached the point where already the common environmental sounds are sufficient to produce auditory perception or the person concerned is at least able to hear his or her own voice. In connection with this last point it is particularly important for the voice to be heard without an ear trumpet since it makes the voice sound quite different,

Lack of autophony in auditory disease

usually much more muffled and hollow. When the deaf person practices listening to his own voice without an ear trumpet the advantage is that he hears his voice mostly by air conduction and only slightly or not at all by bone conduction. When we plug the external auditory meatus in normally hearing individuals their own voice sounds unpleasantly loud and it has a strange quality. This is also the case in lesions involving the sound conducting mechanism. But this so-called autophony does not occur in lesions of the auditory nerve, i.e. with most deaf mutes. Instead, the sound waves are able to produce auditory sensation only by way of the external canal. Therefore, the deaf individual does not hear his own voice at all when the canal is plugged let alone louder which is usually the case in normal hearing.

I exploit this condition for special training of the individual ear. In the case of unsymmetrical hearing in both ears I sometimes have the person listening to his own voice put his finger in his better ear in order to exercise the worse hearing ear particularly.

Special exercises

Results of auditory training

At present I cannot assess the outcome of auditory training because the period of observation has not been long enough and there are relatively few cases that have completed instruction. I must, therefore, limit my discussion to particular points of view.

In addition to the method and manner in which auditory training is practiced the result thereof depends on the state of the hearing and on the personal attitude of the subjects to be instructed. First of all we need to consider in individual cases the state of auditory capability existing previous to instruction and the capacity for development of the auditory sense. As I have previously pointed out even in cases where there is an apparent total loss of hearing, sometimes it is possible to arouse a trace of hearing with the help of patience and perseverance, be it only in one ear, thereby opening the way to further development. Existing remnants of hearing can be increased to hearing for tones, from tone hearing to vowel hearing and that again to a hearing for words. For an existing hearing for words a further improvement in hearing can be attained so that in the course of training whole sentences can be understood, first spoken directly into the ear and then at gradually increasing distances. As I have repeatedly seen for myself in cases where it appears that total deafness is initially present systematic auditory training can lead to gradual increases in hearing so that higher and higher levels of hearing are within reach. Nevertheless, in this connection I must especially point out that capacity for development in individual cases appears unpredictable. Even in instances in which the right and left ear are initially functionally equal development in both ears may vary. Thus sometimes auditory development proceeds more rapidly in one ear than in the other or, at other times, is limited to one ear only. It is also possible that only after a more or less significant improvement in one ear the other ear becomes gradually accessible to positive development. While in many cases higher and higher hearing levels are attained relatively rapidly others remain at a lower level and seem to be temporarily or permanently inaccessible to further hearing development.

A brilliant example of what goal-oriented procedure and patient dedication can accomplish is the work of the lower Austrian State School for the Deaf in Döbling (Vienna); the results with 60 pupils acoustically trained for half a year follow:

TABLE 1. DATA ON INSTRUCTED CHILDREN
Lower Austrian School for the Deaf Vienna, 27 April 1894

	Sentence Hearing	Word Hearing	Vowel Hearing	Some remnants of hearing unquestionable total deafness	Total
II Cl. Teacher *Baldrian*, 12 pupils Hearing capability—start		1	4	7	12
Hearing capability—end (Since 1893 irregularly taught several times a week for five minutes)	4	6	2		
II Cl. Teacher *Bürklen*, 13 pupils Hearing capability—start		1	4	8	13

TABLE 1. DATA ON INSTRUCTED CHILDREN

	Sentence Hearing	Word Hearing	Vowel Hearing	Some remnants of hearing unquestionable total deafness	Total
Hearing capability—end		4	4	5	
III Cl. Teacher *Müller*, 3 pupils					
Hearing capability—start			2	1	3
Hearing capability—end (Since 1893 irregularly taught)		1	2		
III Cl. Teacher *Merkle*, 2 pupils					
Hearing capability—start			1	1	2
Hearing capability—end (Taught since October, 1893)		2			
IV Cl. Teacher *Czerny*, 2 pupils					
Hearing capability—start			1	1	2
Hearing capability—end (Irregularly taught since Oct.)	1	1			
IV Cl. Teacher *Güntschl*, 4 pupils					
Hearing capability—start			2	2	4
Hearing capability—end (Irregularly taught since 1893)		2	2		

TABLE 1. DATA ON INSTRUCTED CHILDREN

	Sentence Hearing	Word Hearing	Vowel Hearing	Some remnants of hearing unquestionable total deafness	Total
V Cl. Teacher J. *Kraft*, 6 pupils					
Hearing capability—start		2	4		6
Hearing capability—end	4	2			
(Irregularly taught since 1893)					
VI Cl. Director *Lehfeld*, 13 pupils					
Hearing capability—start		2	2	9	13
Hearing capability—end	4		5	4	
(Taught for 3 months)					
VIII Cl. Teacher *Kühnel*, 5 pupils					
Hearing capability—start			2	3	5
Hearing capability—end	3	1	1		
(Taught since Sept., 1893)					
Total					60

A summary of the 60 cases follows:

	At start of training	After 6 months
Hearing remnants	32 pupils	11 pupils
Vowel hearing	22	21
Word hearing	6	16
Sentence hearing	0	12
	60	60

The following remarks may serve to explain this table:

All cases of vowel hearing advanced to word hearing and in addition 6 cases advanced to sentence hearing to which 6 cases progressed from their original category making 12 cases in all which advanced to sentence hearing; there remain 16 cases with word hearing; among these 6 which originally had word hearing and 12 which had progressed to that point (28 cases in all) 12 advanced to sentence hearing and 16 fell into the word hearing category. Thirty-two cases started out showing some remnants of hearing. Of these 11 were not ostensibly improved while the remaining 21 progressed to vowel hearing, while the 22 original cases with vowel hearing progressed to a more advanced level of hearing the 21 finally remaining in the vowel hearing group were all only from the remnants-of-hearing category.

These results should be valued all the more highly because they were achieved in a school situation where the instruction time for individual pupils was limited. Actually a large number of them did not even have daily lessons but were instructed every 2–3 days for sessions that were quite short (5–10 minutes).

In the school year 1894–95 the following advances through auditory training took place[115]:

1. From almost total deafness to hearing for sound __ 9 cases
   From almost total deafness to hearing for tones ___ 17 cases
   From almost total deafness to hearing for vowels __ 18 cases
   From almost total deafness to hearing for words __ 4 cases
2. From hearing for sound to hearing for vowels _____ 7 cases
   From hearing for sound to hearing for words _____ 2 cases
3. From hearing for tones to hearing for vowels _____ 2 cases
   From hearing for tones to hearing for words _____ 3 cases
   From hearing for tones to hearing for sentences __ 2 cases

4. From hearing for vowels to hearing for words _____ 9 cases

From hearing for vowels to hearing for sentences _ <u>9</u> cases

Total for instructed cases 92

Since it should also be of interest to report observations on the value of auditory training with the deaf from another source, I present the following report of Instructor to the Deaf *Bestič* in Agram[116].

"In relation to the time I had at my disposal for such activity and given the means at my disposal, namely my speech, five small bells of various frequencies designated with the vowels /u/, /a/, /o/, /e/, /I/, a viola and a whistle, no phenomenal results were achieved but at least they are results. What I have observed and achieved until now in the course of two months of acoustic experimentation with our deaf pupils follows:

1. Of 15 pupils one has been deaf since birth, not a good candidate for acquisition of speech and hence also for this training, but still he hears and differentiates all five vowels.

2. Seven pupils who were totally deaf; four since birth, one lost his hearing in the fifth month, one in the first year and one in his seventh year; they can more or less hear the five vowels and can say them after hearing them. Yet we must shout with all our might if the children are to hear and differentiate among this or that vowel. With the help of a hearing tube the purchase of which was approved by the Ministry of Education, I hope that this result may be accomplished easier and faster.

3. Four pupils, totally deaf as those mentioned above; one lost his hearing in the third month, one in the seventh month, one in the fourth year and the other in the seventh year; at present they are able to hear and discriminate all five vowels and say them after hearing them, besides they are able to identify to a certain degree the tones of the small bells, of the viola and the whistle at a distance of 1–3 decimeters.

4. Of the remaining 4 pupils one is congenitally deaf, one lost his hearing in the first year, the third in the third year and the fourth in the fourth year. One was totally

deaf, the other heard only in one ear the intensely spoken sound / e /, the other two were not completely deaf. Acoustic training with these children now enables them (a) to hear single words and short, familiar, clearly and loudly spoken sentences at a distance from 2 decimeters to 2 meters; (b) to guess at the vowels related to high and low tones of the small bell at a distance of 1–3 decimeters; (c) to track to a certain degree at a distance of 1–2 decimeters the high and low tones of the viola; (d) to differentiate among and to count the number of pips of the whistle at a distance from 1 decimeter to 2 meters.

In my experience to date I have observed that mainly in the beginning exhaustion rapidly occurs followed by a certain nervous fatigue which required interruption of the planned instruction for a shorter or longer time. I noticed, too, that we must undertake training even when it appears that the effort will be fruitless. For example, I first achieved an objective on 2 November which I had originally set for 1 October; with one of the pupils I already thought my labors were in vain, yet on 2 November when I continued the acoustic training as before, I reached the desired result. Now this lad hears all the vowels quite well and, what is more, familiar monosyllabic words which he can repeat after listening to them. Finally, I have also observed that hearing varies. On one day it is keener on another weaker, again on a third it is more acute than on the first. Furthermore, the children do not hear equally well in both ears but sometimes better on the left ear and sometimes in the right ear while it frequently seems to me that they hear only in one ear."

The mental state of the deaf among other things can greatly influence the developmental potential of the auditory sense. The mental capacities of the deaf frequently prove to be quite normal and sometimes they actually reveal a special mental alertness. In other cases mental retardation occurs along with deafness. Furthermore, we need to keep in mind that a deaf mute child, especially of poor parents, often has enjoyed very little education or none at all before it has been handed over to a teacher of the deaf, and enters the school for the deaf intellectually neglected.

Influence of mental state of the deaf on outcome of training

*Attitude of the deaf
towards auditory
training*

It is clear that in such cases we can start acoustic training only after having raised the mental level.*

Not to be underestimated is the attitude of deaf mutes toward auditory training. In the majority of cases the previously unfamiliar sensory experience is very stimulating for the deaf and they bring a great deal of enthusiasm to the training. Later, now and then, especially when progress has been slow and auditory capability has fluctuated markedly, a noticeable disillusion and even discouragement sets in which if combined with complacency and lack of a systematic procedure can easily lead to the abandonment of auditory training. In order to maintain an alert interest it is important also to include in the lessons words that are meaningful to the students but in general to continue the exercises without fail, even if some amount of pressure is required. Just as the confident handling of a musical instrument is possible only through laborious exercises so is the attainment of steadily improved discriminating hearing achieved only through systematic auditory training. The intelligent deaf person soon realizes this. There is the exceptional situation where every attempt to influence hearing by auditory training founders on the indifference or even the aversion of the deaf person to such training. Thus an otherwise mentally alert girl explained to me that she was resigned to her condition and did not want to undergo the annoyance of auditory training.

Practical value of auditory training

The practical value of auditory training is not only its influence on the speech of the deaf mute but also a certain

---

* The present situation in which mentally retarded deaf children are enrolled in schools for the deaf is deplorable both for mentally normal deaf children and the retarded children themselves because obviously both groups cannot be taught in the same way and are therefore bound to hinder each others' progress. So much valuable time of instruction is lost in this way to normal deaf children and so much more productive would their instruction be if the teacher would not simultaneously have to cope with retarded children. For the retarded children themselves, a plan especially suited to these unfortunates would certainly be more productive than is possible in the current situation. We should call particular attention to this persistent flaw in our humanitarian institutions and we should stress that the establishment of special public schools for these children is a pressing need. It is indeed a humanitarian requirement.

the person communicating with the deaf to speak with them by ear rather than by eye since it is difficult for most people to speak with sufficiently conspicuous lip movements to enable the deaf to read them easily."

It is much easier to get into the habit of speaking somewhat louder than usual. Thus, through strengthening of his hearing the deaf person is brought closer to the rest of mankind and society will in turn approach him more willingly if the contact with him is somehow facilitated. Without hearing (as weak as it may be) the deaf person remains isolated from society. A chasm remains which only a partial recovery of hearing can bridge."

Thus, several of the people I have treated who were originally severely or totally deaf obtained employment only because through systematic auditory training they were enabled to hear loudly spoken sentences. Among these cases was the deaf boy who inspired me to embark on my acoustic investigations. This boy who was afflicted with a cleft palate acquired intelligible pronunciation as his hearing improved and after two years of systematic auditory training was able to hear sentences that were spoken moderately loudly into his ear. Four years ago in this state of hearing he entered employment in a book printing shop, initially on a trial basis because the employer wanted to satisfy himself that his hearing was adequate for communication. It was found to be sufficient and the young man has performed his work capably for the last 4 years. The state of his hearing has apparently remained unchanged in recent years.

Deaf mutes who show an even greater capacity for improvement will obviously obtain employment or an occupation all the more easily. This opens a broad rich field for our profession and even if it takes a great deal of sacrifice and labor to cultivate this field, its fruits will give reason for the greatest joy and satisfaction.

Chapter Two

Effect of Systematic Auditory Training on the Sense of Hearing of Those with Acquired Severe Hearing Impairment or Deafness Later in Life

Hyperacusis Willisii

It is a fact known for a long time that many severely hearing-impaired people hear surprisingly better in the presence of noise or during presentation to the ear of varied sound stimuli. This phenomenon is called Hyperacusis or *Paracusis Willisii* since *Willis* (1680) was the first to report such an observation and told of an otherwise deaf woman who heard spoken words only in the presence of drumbeats. *Beck*[119] cites cases where hearing seemed better in the presence of a strong wind, rumbling of a carriage, and claps of thunder. *Fielitz*[120] knew a boy who could hear only in the presence of sole leather being slapped on a stone or during the clatter of a mill. *Politzer*[121] calls attention to the phenomenon that stimulating the bones of the head with tones of tuning forks can result in improved hearing for noises and speech. The possibility of improved hearing in the presence of noise with existing hearing impairment is currently generally known. However, there are still quite varied opinions about the precise nature of such an effect on hearing. Most of the authors, among them *Buck, Bürkner, Politzer, Roosa, Toynbee, Tröltsch, Weber-Liel, Willis,* assume that an increase in hearing in noise is due to an increased improved capacity for vibration of the conductive mechanism especially of the ossicles which occurs as a consequence of intense sound stimulation. In contrast some observers (*Gellé, Löwenberg, Joh Müller, Rau*) take the position that *Hyperacusis Willisii* results from an increase in auditory sensitivity. My observations definitely support the latter opinion especially since I was able to demonstrate that hearing during sound stimulation also increases for persons with normal hearing and that diminution of hearing does not always take place immediately on termination of sound stimulation but that the increased hearing can persist for some time afterward[122].

The main results of my investigations follow[123]: When sound stimulation to a normal ear which hears more poorly in noise is reduced, for example, by plugging the ears the ear can not only maintain its perceptual capacity for a specific sound source but can even show an increase in perception. One and the same noise affects normal-hearing individuals unequally, even one ear more than the other. The effect for rhythmic sound waves (speech, tuning fork) and for non-rhythmic ones (clock, noise) is not always the same. Thus, perception of the clock in noise can appear decreased while it can be increased for speech. The effect of a noise on the auditory function of the hard-of-hearing is much more pronounced. Only in noise are many of them able to experience certain sounds, for example, the ticking of a clock. This can be the case even if the hearing-impaired person does not perceive the noise exciting his auditory function but that noise is very close to his threshold of sensation. The hearing-impaired frequently show an improvement of hearing in noise for

Effect of sound stimulation on the sense of hearing

rhythmic as well as for non-rhythmic sounds, sometimes only for rhythmic ones. Each ear can behave differently even in total contrast to the other. At other times a weak noise has no influence on hearing ability. Individuals with an involvement of the acoustic nerve can also show improved hearing in noise; however, this improvement occurs quite often only at the onset of noise stimulation while subsequently and sometimes very rapidly, hearing ability decreases with continuing noise as a result of auditory fatigue. Similar phenomena are also seen in cases of middle ear involvement and are comparable to nervous asthenia of the eye.

In assessing the nature of improved hearing in noise the decisive fact is that alterations of sound conduction do not always immediately result in change of sound perception. Therefore it can be shown that noises can produce increased perception in unplugged ears of normal hearing persons. Sometimes fading of auditory excitability is remarkably slow; sometimes there even is further increase in excitability after the noise has been interrupted; at other times excitability starts to increase only after the noise has stopped or increase in hearing is preceded by a diminution in hearing. Finally, there are cases where noise stimulation brings about a change for the worse which then slowly recedes, enabling one to trace more exactly the rate of increase in auditory sensitivity.

Tests with various tones of tuning forks show that high tones are more auditorily exciting in general than low ones although there are cases in which one particular tone enhances auditory sensitivity. In some cases noises and vibrations of the body cause improvement in hearing that can last for hours.

Loading the ossicles and the labyrinthine window so that vibration is made impossible or at least much impeded in no way precludes an improvement of hearing in noise. All the experimental results therefore indicate that improved hearing in noise is due to enhanced auditory sensitivity and that any contribution to this phenomenon by the conductive apparatus is doubtful.

In isolated cases the improvement in hearing can last

for a long time after the cessation of sound stimulation. In a most striking instance I observed this in a colleague who after every lengthy train ride (12–16 hours) experienced an improvement in hearing for speech and various sounds for 24 hours[124]. *Kosegarten* mentions cases where bell ringing triggered improvement in hearing for several minutes[125]. The possibility for enhancement of the auditory sense by sound stimulation can be noted from a number of other observations. Thus *Hughes*, as *Brown*[126] reports, found that the use of the audiometer made his ears more sensitive not only for the tones of that instrument but for all environmental noise. In a discussion of the subject *Keown* pointed out that instruction in speech also improves hearing.

Longer lasting improvement in hearing by sound stimulation

According to my observations, even normal hearing is temporarily sharpened by attentive listening and, indeed, not only in the trained but also in the untrained ear. This indicates enhanced excitability of the acoustic centers just as my investigations of monocular vision show that excitation of the optic center results in enhancement of vision in both eyes[127]. The investigations of *Eitelberg*[128] concerning enhancement of hearing yielded similar results.

Effect of acoustic excitation

The careful observer will frequently notice an enhancement of hearing resulting from concentrated listening, sometimes to a surprising degree. Several hearing-impaired people have told me that after attending an opera they understand speech for a few hours better than previously. After a musical evening a hard-of-hearing man detected the swinging pendulum of his clock that he otherwise never heard. The next morning this improvement in hearing was gone. Some hearing-impaired people note that in the theater they experience a gradual improvement in hearing in the course of the performance. One hard-of-hearing woman told me she is able to understand dialogue on the stage only toward the end of the second hour in the theater. This corresponds to the case mentioned previously where a severely hearing-impaired person could not hear his own words at first when he spoke them loudly, later heard some of them and finally heard them quite clearly.

Such an improvement in hearing can, however, be inhibited by various circumstances, either psychological in nature or as a result of acoustic fatigue. Thus, it is a commonly observed phenomenon that hard-of-hearing people, especially those easily excited, can experience a significant exacerbation of their impairment and can in fact temporarily become almost totally deaf when they become conscious of their hearing difficulty in social interaction or in the theater and, depending on the circumstances, they are affected by great agitation or depression. On other occasions even the fear of not hearing well can cause this kind of auditory disturbance. In considering auditory fatigue which was previously discussed in detail, I confine my remarks only to cases which are diametrically opposed to those mentioned above inasmuch as they experience no improvement in hearing during social interaction or in the theater but actually suffer an increase in hearing impairment. That happens especially with sustained, intense, concentrated listening. Allowing for various individual differences the fatigue normally sets in with a rapidity directly proportional to the amount of concentration required. Indeed it is also a daily experience in school where this phenomenon is frequently wrongly perceived and auditory fatigue is interpreted as inattention.

The observations presented here suggest the importance of acoustic stimulation for hearing impairment, however varied its causes may be, nervous or otherwise. In both cases an enhancement of auditory excitability makes an improvement in hearing possible. Either it results in improving the function of a sluggishly responding sense organ or, if the otherwise normally functioning sound perception is inhibited by an involvement of the conductive apparatus, systematic training causes increased sensitivity to weak sound stimuli so that now even a response to pathologically attenuated sound waves becomes possible just as in the case of normal auditory sensitivity, function is enhanced through training. However, in the case of severe impairment or lack of mobility of the conductive apparatus not even systematic auditory training will achieve any noteworthy result because in this situation there is little or no sound conduction to the acoustic nerve.

Obviously enhancement of auditory function through training can last only with methodical application while temporary stimulation can have only temporary effects. Again, with minimal acoustic stimulation an increasing auditory sluggishness sets in which will be ever more pronounced because with severe torpidity of the acoustic nerve fewer and fewer sound waves will be strong enough to cause auditory excitation. Unfortunately, this generally happens with individuals who are either unilaterally deaf or have a different degree of impairment in each ear. They use only the normal or the better ear, and, if the impairment is severe on both sides, tend to withdraw more and more from social interaction which results in increasingly reduced sound stimulation. With increasing neglect of acoustic stimulation the existing weakness of auditory function is exacerbated. As I have already commented in my first report on this subject it is "very likely that in some cases of severe hearing impairment the inactivity of the sense of hearing plays a significant role. In this connection the statement of a witty, intelligent lady from Viennese society was of interest to me. This lady told me that her hearing difficulty increased considerably in the silence of her summer sojourn in the country so that on her return to Vienna in the fall she was able to maintain social contacts only with the greatest effort and self-control. With the return to her busy social life there was a regular gradual improvement in her hearing up to a certain level that has remained almost unchanged for years. I believe that this observation can be associated with inactivity of the auditory sense just as similar observations concerning the significance of inactivity of the visual sense have been well known for a time[129]."

I therefore advise the hard-of-hearing to stimulate their ears as much as possible, in their social contacts as well as through music or theater.* Of great importance

---

*It has been frequently observed that hearing-impaired persons become ill-tempered and discouraged when they are able to follow a performance in the theater only partially. I urge such people to attend the theater diligently not for their pleasure but for auditory training. When there are signs of acoustic fatigue they should relax their attention for a while, and only concentrate again after they have recovered. These people then attend the theater from a quite different standpoint and, as I have often noticed, will not be as easily discouraged by their hearing impairment.

are auditory exercises with speech to be repeated several times daily. Speech should be presented directly to the ear so that lipreading is not possible. Where there is bilateral unsymmetrical hearing impairment the poorer hearing ear should not be neglected but should get special attention[130].

For persons with severe impairment as well as for those with acquired deafness the same auditory training should be instituted as for deaf mutes, also, as previously described, auditory sensitivity is stimulated.

The emergence of speech comprehension through systematic auditory training in individuals who have acquired deafness late in life is sometimes gradual as in the case of the congenitally deaf, sometimes improvement is very rapid so that a person initially deaf to speech hears single words and even sentences sometimes after just a few lessons. This concerns mostly cases where various sound sources (as concertinas, tuning forks, speech sounds) produce a clear, with intense stimulation even uncomfortably strong auditory sensation, but where speech sounds or words shouted into the ear are not understood but generate only a diffuse sensation. If, on the other hand, these people are informed beforehand which sounds and words are to be presented in the speech lessons they usually acquire correct understanding for these speech sounds in a short time, sometimes even when the familiar syllables and words are spoken at some distance from the ear, moderately loud or even in a whisper. At the same time such a person can lack understanding for other words and sentences, especially for those that have not been presented previously. In this connection there are some quite surprising phenomena.

Psychic deafness

Thus, in the case of a deafened French woman who spoke German well, I used that language in the first training sessions and in a few days achieved a significant improvement of her condition to the point where for a number of sentences a normal conversational tone was sufficient for comprehension. One day as I unexpectedly began to speak French to this patient she appeared to be completely deaf to speech in her mother tongue, even to loud words, while she could hear correctly sentences spoken in German at a moderate level, among them some which had not been included in previous instruction. Then, however, only a short time was required to develop comprehension of French speech and to advance quite rapidly. The same observation was reported by my assistant, Dr. *Panzer.* This concerned a Russian lady who spoke German well and whose deafness for German speech receded quickly with instruction employing that language while the first attempt in Russian showed a continuing deafness for it. In such cases a certain kind of psychic deafness appears to be present similar to that found in childhood which, as has been shown, can also develop later in life[131].

Till now I have observed acquired psychic deafness in cases of lues, also following influenza, typhus and due to unknown causes, in nervous as well as in otherwise healthy and robust individuals. This sensory deafness either appeared right away in character, growing gradually stronger—similar to a progressive hearing impairment—or else occured suddenly, after preceding fluctuations in hearing in which case it was interpreted as nervously induced deafness. This disturbance in hearing, I believe, has been up to now incorrectly diagnosed in adults. It is different from other nervous involvement inasmuch as it is caused by a simple functional disturbance of the sense organ in the presence of an otherwise partially or completely intact conductive pathway. These cases in which auditory exercises produce rapid improvement in hearing indicate the presence of specific functional disorders of auditory perception rather than that of destructive processes.

Finally, I should discuss an interesting phenomenon which occurs when we undertake systematic auditory training with persons who acquired deafness later in life, i.e. with those who possessed normal hearing for speech previous to its loss, as compared to deaf mutes who never—or only in early childhood—had hearing for speech. While the congenitally deaf in developing hearing for speech perceive only very slowly articulated syllables and later words, the person who acquired deafness later in life often hears a rapidly spoken word better than one which is slowly called into the ear. This was the case, for example for a man, age 32, who was totally deafened at age 28. When in

Better comprehension of rapid speech (by those who became deaf later in life)

the course of training the sentence "Leiden Sie öfter an Kopfschmerzen?" (Do you have headaches frequently?) was spoken at a slow drawn out rate it was heard as "Leise, s, öfters, heute, weiters." When the question was spoken more rapidly at the same distance from the ear and with the same intensity it was quite correctly heard. The results were confirmed by tests using other sentences.

Combining in listening

We can often make such observations which suggest that a person who has acquired almost total deafness for speech later in life can more easily recognize a partially understood word when it is spoken in the more rapid manner familiar to him prior to his deafness, because it better enables the individual to add parts of words or sentences which were not heard, to the heard parts, while slow speech where syllable follows syllable is more confusing for the combination effort. On the other hand in auditory training employing speech the deaf mute person gets first of all an auditory impression of single phonemes and then has to construct the proper word from the slowly presented single sounds. Accordingly, he is drilled more for this kind of hearing. However, as he progresses in auditory training the deaf person too, learns to combine efficiently.

Only closer scrutiny can indicate what a significant, sometimes unexpectedly major role combination can play in cases of deficient hearing for words. Even the normal-hearing person in everyday conversation by no means hears every sound of a nevertheless clearly understood word. Without being aware of it he fills in the missing sounds according to the sense of the word or sentence. Therefore the hearing of complex sentences is auditorily less demanding than the perception of single words or especially of isolated syllables. A young man tested by me on this point could unhesitatingly repeat sentences spoken moderately loud at a distance of seven paces and could correctly answer different questions put to him at this distance. Yet he was not able to understand a single word with certainty, even when I articulated this word clearly and slowly quite close to his ear. Thus, for example, the words Rand (rim), Sand (sand), Band (string), Land (land), Tand (trifle), Pfand (pledge) were always heard rather unsurely and were con-

fused with one another. He had special difficulty discriminating among the initial consonants which could be demonstrated clearly by presenting the consonants individually.
However, the subject always repeated the word correctly
if it was presented in the context of other words as part
of a sentence. This is easy to understand, e.g. if in the
sentence "Dieses Land ist fruchtbar" (this land is fertile)
the L in the word "Land" would not be correctly heard,
the L would unconsciously be inserted according to the
sense of the sentence. In fact normally a word in a sentence
is easily confused with a similar sounding word if that word
also fits the sentence, but not when it does not fit.

Similar phenomena occur in vision where a whole
object is correctly seen though details of the object may be
unconsciously neglected or again filled in correctly.

APPENDIX

Reports of Cases

In the following I present brief abstracts of the records of individual cases in which systematic auditory training was undertaken.

Cases of Congenital Deafness (Deafmutism)*

1. Josef Kuntner, age 15, student in Class 8 of the Lower Austrian State School for the Deaf, totally deafened by meningitis at the age of 4. Training of the apparently completely deaf boy began on 15 September 1893 and consisted of daily sessions of 10 minutes each continually to 1 December, 1893 with the following results: Both ears heard with absolute certainty the vowels / a /, / e /, / I /, / o /, / u /, the diphthongs / av /, / ɔI /, / aI /, the consonants f, s, b, p, m, n, w, v, r, t, d and about 100 words formed from these sounds. In April, 1894 the lad could recognize all sounds in both ears and had reached a point where he could hear words, sentences and also his own voice.

---

*Cases 1, 2, and 3 were presented to the Society of Clinical Medicine of Vienna on 1 December, 1893 and on 27 April, 1894 (see Wiener Klinische Wochenschrift, 1894, No. 1, 19 and 20)

2. Theresia Hagleitner, age 16, student in Class 8, totally deaf from birth. Since September 15, 1893, training for this girl consisted of 20-minute daily instructional sessions and after 10 weeks she heard the sounds reported for case one, plus / k / and / g /. Since instruction was mostly concentrated on one ear and consequently during almost all of the instructional time this ear (the left) had the advantage, it resulted in a significantly greater acquisition of vocabulary than for case one. The girl eventually understood with certainty sentences and questions which could be presented in context whereas case one heard only single words spoken into the ear. Her other right ear was intentionally minimally stimulated in order to prove that only by systematic training can one make the ear responsive to acoustic stimuli. But in order to meet the possible objection that the hearing results on the right ear were not obtainable at all Instructor *Kühnel* worked preliminarily with the right ear for a four week period using vowels. After this period the right ear perceived these sounds as clearly as the left ear. However, the right ear still did not understand words that the left ear heard clearly. In April, 1894 the girl demonstrated word and sentence hearing, heard her own voice and already understood simple conversation.

3. Walter Küntzel, age 7 from Liebau in Russia, since September, 1893 a boarder with the family of Instructor Kühnel. The boy was deafened eight months previously as a result of cerebrospinal meningitis and was already showing great impairment of pronunciation. At the beginning of auditory training the lad showed total deafness in his right ear, in the left ear he heard only single vowels, and these for the most part incorrectly. On December 1, 1893 he was able with the exclusively trained left ear to hear and to repeat correctly moderately loud sentences spoken at a distance of 50 Cm. When the talker was visible to him the boy was quite able to repeat what was said at a distance up to one meter because in this situation his attention was much more engaged than when he only heard but did not see the talker. Lipreading could not have been involved here because it had not been taught and even if it had been, such facility in lipreading could not be achieved in the short period of two months. Noteworthy, too, is that during the period of auditory training the lad's pronunciation gradually became almost perfect. He received systematic auditory training for half an hour twice a day and in the course of the day received diligent acoustic exposure from various members of the family. In April, 1894 the boy heard speech in his left ear at a distance of up to two meters and could be taught aurally in the various school subjects. While in December, 1893 hearing was stimulated only in the left ear which had been trained exclusively, hearing in the right ear improved steadily after training of that ear had been initiated.

4. This case concerns a 12 year old deaf mute girl, Selma P. who came to me in April, 1895, and was referred for systematic auditory training to Instructor *Kolar* of the Lower Austrian School for the Deaf. During the period from 19 April to 11 July I repeated checked her hearing status. Her record as reported by Her *Kolar* follows.

Initial results based on test with the concertina: Uncertain perception of tones f and g in the left ear and complete impairment of auditory perception in the right ear. Of the tones tested with tuning forks only the left ear was sensitive to a contra-a. Immediately, presentation of the vowels / a / and / I / was begun, at first to the left ear. In the first week discrimination between these sounds was achieved. In the second week / u / and the dipthongs / av / and / aI / were added to the repertoire. In order to thoroughly reinforce elementary vowel hearing in the left ear the following exercises were carried out:

Hearing the vowels separated by intervals / a / / a / / a /
Hearing the vowels in different sequences / a // I /, / I // a /, / u // I // a /
Counting repeated presentations of the same vowel
Differentiation of mere aspiration from the voiced vowel
Introduction of the second sound in diphthongs
Varying duration of vowels

In the following weeks semi-vowels and fricative sounds were practiced. As soon as possible these were combined into words: Aar (eagle), Uhr (watch), Auf (on), Schau (look). After drills on characteristic acoustic qualities of all vowels and consonants elementary words and syllables were employed, for example, ba (interjection), ab (off), Bau (building), Schaf (sheep), Schuh (shoe), da (there), du (you), Bub (boy), Papa (Daddy), Fass (barrel), Fuss (foot), der, die, das (determinate articles). Then after some acoustical word patterns for the purpose of auditory discrimination were remembered words to be used were grouped according to the main vowels. The choice was based on *Vatter's* Primer. For example, A-group: ba (interj.), ab (off), Papa (daddy), Fass (barrel), brav (nice), Aff (ape), Schaf (sheep), das (that), Aas (carrion). For repetition the nouns were practiced with the article. In a similar way the remaining sound groups were presented. Then the most frequently occurring consonant clusters were given in their natural sequence just as they occur in spelling and reading instruction. It was now possible to practice short sentences. First, various simple ones: Pass auf! (Pay attention) Papa ist brav. (Daddy is nice) Bist du brav?(Are you nice?)

It should be noted that the material presented up to now was aimed only at the left ear. There were problems with the right ear and only after a month of training was the exact differentiation of the primary vowels / a / / i / / u / achieved and the most important consonants introduced.

Gradually the auditory capability of the right ear increased and after two months of training the same drill material could be used for both ears. The left ear is more advanced inasmuch as it is also trained in hearing at a distance. For the time being drills in this ear concentrate on concertina tones, simple vowels and the diphthongs.

To contribute to accurate discrimination of words, the same sentence is spoken with varying word order. For example, Der Papa ist brav. (Daddy is nice) Ist der Papa brav? (Is daddy nice?) Brav ist der Papa! (Nice is daddy) These sentences should be especially chosen to stimulate the child's interest and participation.

Materials conveniently at hand should first be employed in training. Among these are items constituting general classes such as parts of the body—Leib (body), Fuss (foot), Arm (arm), Ohr (ear), Haar (hair) etc., articles of clothing, colors, etc., drill on question and answer: Wie ist? (How is?), Wo ist? (Where is?), Was ist? (What is?) Wie alt bist du? (How old are you?), Wie heisst du? (What is your name?). The principle is that new words should be perceived exclusively by hearing.

After thorough training and correct auditory discrimination of these elementary questions, questions and statements related to daily living based on *Lehfeld's* "Lehrbuch der Umgangssprache" (Textbook of colloquial speech) should be practiced. Thus, included would be days of the week and related questions, the organization of the face of the clock, the weather, the seasons, the months of the year, the compass directions, the names of several cities, numerals, also the little words *ma*! ('times' in multiplication), und (and), and the execution of simple operations in arithmetic by ear, etc.

It should be mentioned here that it is very advantageous now and then to include nonsensical and unexpected questions and statements—for example, 'Is the sheep blue'? or to change word order. This contributes much to the total concentration of attention on the sense of hearing. A conceptual complex can be used so that individual sentences will be heard in a context. During repeated drills it is nevertheless advisable to speak in an unorganized manner so that the words will be discriminated exclusively by hearing. It goes without saying that in all of this the teacher must be careful to articulate properly, with attention to such features as varying vowel duration etc. for it is also an important goal of auditory training to develop and improve articulation and voice quality of our deaf children. When in our first classes we introduced auditory exercises for the first time in conjunction with speech instruction we were successful in achieving clear vowels.

To achieve acute hearing, it is also useful to repeat certain words and phrases often in the course of conversation, for example: "Pass auf!" (pay attention), "Selma!", "Ist das wahr?" (Is it true?)

The concertina proved most useful during instruction. When certain tones were played for the first time, they caused a tickling sensation in the ear. Later this feeling subsided and the tones were heard separately.

I have cited this report at length in order to describe the course of training taken in this case in greater detail. I must emphasize that in this case the reported results were achieved after approximately three months of training and, of course, the auditory training is being continued on a regular basis.

Cases of Deafness Acquired Later in Life

1. Ferdinand Schwabl, age 32, in June, 1892 experienced a continuous ringing in the left ear which was accompanied by quick permanent loss of hearing in that ear; a year later the same symptoms appeared without known cause in the right ear. Months of the continual treatment consisting of catheterization and dilation of the tubes yielded no result. At examination on 27 April 1894 the patient appeared to be totally deaf to speech, could not perceive the lower tones of tuning forks at all and the high tones only marginally.

30 April. In the beginning single vowels spoken loudly into the right ear are not heard at all and after a few minutes only incorrectly. Within ten minutes the patient is able to discriminate /a/ and /o/ and is even able to repeat short words correctly. Patient is now advised to undertake auditory exercises for an hour each day preliminarily only on the right ear. In addition I train him three times weekly for 10–15 minutes.

1 May. Except for / e / all vowels are correctly recognized and also single words but / m /, / n /, / s /, / ts /, / f /, / pf / are not heard.

18 May. Patient hears his own loud voice with increasing clarity.

23 May. / e / can still not be discriminated from / I /, except once when whispered sharply into the ear.

25 May. / e / and / I / are by now well discriminated but not / v /, / m /, / n /. Otherwise understanding for speech progresses to the point where short sentences spoken moderately loud close to the ear are understood.

1 June. Tests of the left ear which up to this date had not been trained show that it does not appear to be as deaf as at the beginning of auditory training but can hear all vowels clearly, also words spoken loudly into the ear which are not heard when the left ear is blocked. From now on the left ear is also being trained individually.

11 June. Understanding for speech continues to progress so that the patient who is employed in a large office and who up to a short time previously was not able to understand anyone is now already able to understand a number of his colleagues when they speak directly into his ear.

3 July. Words and sentences spoken loudly are heard at a distance of one meter. At this stage patient understands all 30 colleagues in his office.

8 July. Sharp whispered voice is by and large well understood.

November. Loud to moderately loud sounds were perceived at a distance of two meters.

January to July, 1895. During this entire period the patient has practiced 1–2 hours daily and we can talk with him in a normal conversational tone at 2–3 paces. The initial uncertainty in understanding single words is almost completely gone by July. The hearing still shows slow improvement.

2. Hermine T., age 15½, measles at the age of 6, followed by bilateral clouding of the cornea and blindness. These, however, were due to a hereditary lues involvement. With antisyphilitic treatment sight returned completely. At age 7, ostensibly after a cold, a progressive hearing impairment appeared in both ears. Despite ventilation, 49 pilocarpin injections and an electrical treatment this turned into total deafness for speech which had remained unchanged for the last five years before I began auditory training with the girl. On 27 June 1894 hearing tests showed total deafness for speech in both ears so that even vowels shouted loudly into the ear were not heard; however, there was perception for various tones of tuning forks.

27 June. Within a quarter of an hour vowels are pretty well discriminated in the stimulated left ear.

28 June. 2–3 digit numbers spoken loudly into the ear are to some extent correctly heard.

4 July. The left ear hears short sentences, also and the right which has been stimulated for several days.

13. July. Sentences spoken moderately loudly close to the ear are heard completely by the left ear, somewhat less well by the right ear.

July-November. Hearing gradually improves even for musical tones which are not included in the instruction. The girl who is employed as a supernumerary in a theater has a fine opportunity in her position to convince herself of her gradually improving hearing. While she was formerly totally deaf to various sound sources she began to hear orchestral music, initially as noise, then individual tones and finally these in their melodic configurations. In a similar manner, loud voices on the stage at first generated confused auditory sensations. In the course of weeks the girl recognized single speech sounds and here and there a word.

19 November. The tones of a barrel-organ are heard for the first time and simultaneously the rhythm of the waltz is recognized.

2 January 1895. Patient hears singing for the first time at a distance of one pace. A progressive improvement in hearing for speech is noted so that an increasing number of persons is understood.

January to July. Understanding for speech progresses further; on some days normal conversation is heard at a distance of ½ meter. Also in the theater the girl notes a progressive improvement in hearing for music and is able to hear the musical pieces played by the orchestra. Patient now also understands individual words and sentences spoken on the stage. Hearing is still getting slowly and steadily better.

In addition, it is worthy of note that within the first six months of training the girl forgot her lip-reading. The patient had mastered lipreading on advice from another source but had strict orders from me right from the inception of auditory training not to depend on the eye but during training to rely exclusively on the ear. I generally advise against lipreading as long as there is still a possibility for development of hearing because lipreading has an adverse effect on independent hearing.

3. Bertha Kl., age 25, except for smallpox at age 5 and diphtheria in childhood with resulting permanent paralysis of the pupillary sphincter of the right eye had been in good health to the end of December, 1891. In January, 1892 she suddenly experienced headache, vertigo and vomiting which lasted for a month. At the end of February she became ill ostensibly from influenza of the catarrhal variety. On 8 March patient noted a tinnitus and diminution of hearing in her right ear. She sought treatment which continued with interruptions, and till June, 1893 improved the condition of her hearing impairment and tinnitus.

On 26 July, 1893 while working as a cashier, patient suddenly experienced bilateral total deafness without any other associated symptoms. It was diagnosed as acoustic anaesthesia and in October-November a series of pilocarpin injections was administered without result. Patient heard only once during this treatment, when the word "Mutter!" (mother) was shouted into her ear. Later she underwent galvanic treatment which was repeated 50 times (in the months of December, 1893 and January, 1894). After this treatment, too, was without result and when on occasion of another consultation her condition was diagnosed as incurable acoustic anaesthesia* the patient discontinued all treatment. I saw her for the first time on 27 March 1894. The examination showed an almost total anaesthesia of the acoustic nerve. Low, middle and high tones of tuning forks are barely detected by air or bone conduction. Various musical tones do not give rise to the slightest auditory sensation. Thus, the patient is deaf to the piano and zither as well as other string instruments and does not even hear the loudest martial or orchestral music. Furthermore, patient appears deaf to speech in both ears and shows only slight traces of hearing with loud shouting in the right or left ear, somewhat more on the right ear than the left. Examination of the external and middle ear shows no detectable pathology except for negligible clouding of both tympanic membranes.*

*When I presented this patient to the scientific congress in Vienna in September, 1894 Professor *Politzer* commented that, as far as he recalled, the patient who was known to him had temporarily

Immediately on the first day the patient was presented to me, on 27 March, I began auditory training of the kind I employ with deaf mutes and continued the instruction for 10–15 minutes daily; in addition patient was instructed in the same way by various people around her, so that since 27 March total daily training amounted to an hour per day. The result was striking, for after three days of instruction single words were already heard in the exclusively trained right ear but the various voices sounded muffled and hollow. This strange interference disappeared slowly in the course of the next two weeks while the hearing progressed quite impressively so much so that in the third week patient already understood sentences spoken loudly into the right ear. Only certain phonemes and syllables were heard faintly or not at all, especially on some days. Special exercises had to be instituted with these sounds. In speaking whole sentences, particularly in a loud voice, a curious phenomenon appeared, namely that the patient heard the voice as suddenly very high-pitched. This subjective increase in pitch occurred equally with a high or a low voice but gradually diminished in the course of a few months. After a month of training patient was able to hear complete sentences spoken into her right ear, on some days already sharply whispered speech. She also began to repeat correctly sentences spoken loudly from a distance of ½ m to 1 m. A particularly rapid increase in improvement in hearing occurred in the fourth week of instruction. In the course of the years 1894 and 1895 hearing improvement progressed slowly. Patient is now able to hear normal conversational tone when spoken up close and directed to the ear. Moderately loud speech is understood at a distance of one to two paces; noticeable also is a steady improvement in hearing for music. Training is continuing.

---

regained her hearing after her deafness occurred, and that it was doubtful in this case whether the improvement in hearing could be attributed to auditory training since recovery could also have been spontaneous. To counter this I need to mention that according to recent inquiries, including that of the patient's mother, I was positively assured that fluctuations in the hearing of the patient were observed only at the beginning of her ear involvement, but that total deafness had persisted from its sudden onset on 26 July 1893 to the inception of my auditory training (27 March 1894), that is, for eight months.

Finally, I must emphasize that there is no history of nervous involvement in the family of the patient nor does she present any nervous symptoms. There seems to be no basis in this case for a presumed hypothesis of hysterically caused acoustic anaesthesia.

4. Pasqualina O. from Odessa, 40 years old, came to me for treatment in July, 1895. Fifteen years ago as a result of typhus patient had been totally deafened in the left ear and severely hearing-impaired in the right ear. In the course of several years, ventilation, electrical therapy and pilocarpin yielded no improvement and so the patient abandoned all treatment. Then, a few years after treatment had been terminated there was a spontaneous increase in hearing in both ears, particularly in the right ear in which she now heard normally nine years after overcoming typhus. However, the patient felt otherwise weak and easily irritated. The good hearing in the right ear remained unchanged for five years. Suddenly in August, 1894 without any known cause total deafness appeared in the right ear which persisted for several days, then turned into severe hearing impairment, then again to complete deafness. These fluctuations in hearing were manifest for ten days. At the same time the patient suffered spasms and shivering of the entire body. Ten days after the onset of deafness the fluctuations ceased. From then on patient was totally deaf to speech and was able to perceive only single sounds. Therapy directed at the hysterical symptoms including hydropathic procedures resulted in a definite improvement in hearing as such but not for understanding of speech that seemed to be irretrievably lost. Patient experienced a feeling of pressure in the head, headache, vertigo and intense tinnitus (buzzing and humming).

On 13 July 1895 my examination of both ears of this otherwise healthy and robust looking patient yielded no significant findings in the external or middle ears. The hearing test showed total bilateral deafness for speech, whereas hearing for all concertina tones as well as for tuning fork sounds appeared to be quite normal. As a matter of fact when the patient was stimulated more intensely with these sounds she always started with fright and indicated that she was experiencing a painful sensation in the ears and head. The same phenomenon occurred with speech sounds, but they were not understood.

13 July. After several minutes of auditory exercises patient understands not only the vowels but also words and even short sentences, eventually including words that were called into her ear for the first time. Patient is advised to have friends and family take part in her auditory training. On 17 July after just four days of instruction patient was already able to hear and, for the most part, to understand correctly entire conversations that took place very loudly close to her ear. She was even able to understand digits whispered into her ear as well as moderately loud sentences although not always correctly. At the end of July when I left Vienna a steady increase in understanding of speech was evident so that at that time slow conversation conducted at a distance half a pace from the ear could be correctly repeated including single words. My assistant Dr. *Panzer*, who continued the training, informed me at the time when I finished this study (mid-August) that there was further improvement in the hearing for speech so that at present we can carry on colloquial conversation at a normal rate and volume close to the ear. Furthermore, Dr. *Panzer* reported to me as follows: "One day I suddenly began speaking Russian to the patient without alerting her beforehand. Russian is her mother tongue. Despite the fact that I spoke unusually loud and that finally I practically screamed single words into her ear she understood nothing at first. Only after a lengthy time of continued instruction did she gradually recognize her mother tongue and was able to understand what she heard."

Reference Notes

1. Majer, E.H. Zur Geschichte der HNO-Heilkunde in Österreich. *Laryngol. Rhinol. Otol.* 7:406–411 (1980).
2. Perelló, J. *The History of International Association of Logopedics and Phoniatrics.* Editorial, Augusta, S.A., Barcelona, 1976.
3. Bezold, F. Das Hörvermögen der Taubstummen. Verlag von J.F. Bergmann, Wiesbaden, 1896.
4. Lincke, Handbuch der Ohrenheilkunde (Otology). 1845, II, p. 11.
5. Ibid. p. 17.
6. Ibid. p. 23.
7. Académie des sciences de Paris, 1768, V, p. 500.
8. Traité des maladies de l'oreille, 1821, II p. 474–492.
9. Deuxiéme circulaire de l'Institut des sourds-muets de Paris, 1829, p. 36.
10. Boyer, La Voix, Paris 1895, VI, Nr. 61, p. 12, 13.
11. Bericht über die Taubstummen-Anstalt in Bern, 1823–1824.
12. Die Krankheiten des Gehörorganes, 1827, p. 36.
13. Stuttgart, 1830.
14. Ohrenheilkunde, 1845, p. 418.
15. Ohrenheilkunde. English (Toynbee) original, 1860. German translation by Moos, 1863, p. 416–421.
16. See the paper by Boyer, La Voix, 1895, VI, No. 61.
17. Revue internationale de l'enseignement de sourds-muets, January, 1892.
18. 13. Jahresbericht der Niederösterreichischen Landes-Taubstummenschule in Döbling-Wien, 1894, p. 6. (Thirteenth annual report of the Lower Austrian State School for the Deaf).
19. Wiener klinische Wochenschrift 1893, No. 29; Vortrag (Lecture) in der k.k. Gesellsch.d.Aertze (Physicians) in Wien, 1 December, 1893 (Wiener klinische Wochenschrift 1894, No. 1 and 27 April, 1894 (Wiener klinische Wochenschrift 1894, No. 19 and 20).
20. Sitzung (meeting) der k.k. Gesellschaft der Aerzte in Wien, 27 April, 1894.
21. Bericht der 3. deutschen Taubstummenlehrer-Versammlung in Augsburg, 1894, p. 121. (Proceedings of the third congress of teachers of the deaf, Augsburg, 1894).
22. Ibid. p. 129.
23. Ibid. p. 126.

24. Wiener klinische Wochenschrift July, 1893.
25. Agramer Zeitung 10 November, 1893.
26. See also Goldstein (St. Louis) Arch. of Otology, 1895, XXIV, No. 1.
27. Berlin, 1895.
28. Lincke, Handbuch der Ohrenheilkunde, 1845, III, p. 223.
29. Pflüger's Archiv, 1883, XXXI, p. 284.—Archiv für Ohrenheilkunde, 1893, XXXV, p. 15.
30. Pflüger's Archiv, 1883, XXXI, p. 280.
31. Ibid. p. 303.
32. Pflügers Archiv für Physiologie 1881, XXV, p. 325.
33. See also Toynbee, p. 419.
34. Ohrenheilkunde. Translated, 183, p. 419.
35. Münchener medizinische Wochenschrift 1893, No. 48.
36. Archiv für Ohrenheilkunde. 1867, II, p. 268.
37. Knapp, Archiv für Augen-und Ohrenheilkunde 1871, II, Abtheilung 1, p. 291.
38. Horns Archiv, 1859, I, p. 8.
39. Phil. Transact. 1820, p. 306. See Archiv für Physiologie 1823, VIII, p. 413 and Schmidts Jahrbuch CXX, p. 246.
40. Ref. 8, 48.
41. Heidelberger natur wissenschaftlich-medizinische Verhandlungen, 6 December, 1861. See also Moos, Klinik der Ohrenheilkunde, 1866, p. 36.
42. Virchows Archiv 1864, XXXI, p. 125.
43. Archiv für Ohrenheilkunde III, p. 136.
44. Zeitschrift für Ohrenheilkunde III, p. 174.
45. Archiv für Augen-und Ohrenheilkunde, 1871, II, p. 276, 279, 290, 317.
46. Archiv für Ohrenheilkunde, XXI, p. 300.
47. Arch.f.Augen-u.Ohrenheilkunde, IV, p. 125. Zeitschrift für Ohrenheilkunde, XX, p. 203.
48. Cf. Politzer, Ohrenheilkunde 2 Auflage, p. 481.
49. Ohrenheilkunde 1889, 4 Auflage, p. 56.
50. Zeitschrift für Ohrenheilkunde XX, p. 200.
51. Archiv für Ohrenheilkunde XXXII, p. 53 and XXXV, p. 299.
52. Deutsche medizinische Wochenschrift 1889, Centralbl. für Physiologie 1889, No. 15.
53. Compt. rend. May 1845. Cf. Lincke-Wolff, Ohrenheilkunde III, p. 114.
54. Archiv für Augen und Ohrenheilkunde IV, Abtheilung 1, p. 165.
55. Archiv für Ohrenheilkunde XV, p. 273.
56. Archiv für Ohrenheilkunde XXX, p. 1.
57. Archiv für Ohrenheilkunde XXII, p. 177.
58. Zeitschrift für Ohrenheilkunde X, p. 1.
59. Virchows Archiv, XCIV.
60. Archiv für Ohrenheilkunde 1888, p. 85.
61. Monatsschrift für Ohrenheilkunde 1888, p. 85.
62. Archiv für Ohrenheilkunde XXX, p. 1.
63. Zeitschrift für Heilkunde, X u. XII.
64. Burckhardt-Merian, Archiv für Ohrenheilkunde XXII, p. 177.
65. Zeitschrift für Ohrenheilkunde XXIV, p. 267.
66. Academie der Wissenschaften, Berlin, May, 1881; June 1883; February, 1886.

67. Zeitschrift für Ohrenheilkunde X, p. 1.
68. Archiv für Ohrenheilkunde XVI, p. 171.
69. Archiv für Ohrenheilkunde XXVII, p. 105.
70. Schwartzes Handbuch der Ohrenheilkunde II, p. 513.
71. Burckhardt-Merian, Archiv für Ohrenheilkunde XXII, p. 177.
72. Archiv für Augen-und Ohrenheilkunde II, Abth. 2, p. 64.
73. Archiv für Ohrenheilkunde III, p. 198.
74. Zeitschrift für Ohrenheilkunde XXII, p. 285.
75. Politzer, Archiv für Ohrenheilkunde I, p. 70; Mach and Kessel, Akademie der Wissenschaften, Wien, 1872, cf. Archiv für Ohrenheilkunde VIII, p. 90; Shapringer, Akademie der Wissenschaften, Wien, LXXII; Blake and Shaw, cf. Archiv für Augen-und Ohrenheilkunde III, p. 209.
76. Archiv für Ohrenheilkunde I, p. 316; III, p. 202.
77. Archiv für Ohrenheilkunde XIV, p. 1.
78. Cf. Beck, Krankheiten des Gehörorganes, 1827, p. 237.
79. Horns Archiv, 1859, I, p. 8.
80. Internationaler Medizinischer Congress, Berlin, 1890.
81. Cf. Schmidts Jahrbuch 1863, CXX, p. 246.
82. Archiv der physiologischen Heilkunde, 1847, p. 447.
83. Über Störungen der musikalischen Leistungsfähigkeit bei Gehirnläsion, Inaug.-Dissert., Leipzig, 1888 (Disburbances of musical perception in lesions of the brain); Deutsches Archiv für klinische Medizin XLIII, p. 331, Archiv für Psychologie XX.
84. Der aphasische symptomencomplex (The symptom complex in aphasia). Breslau, 1874.
85. Wiener klinische Wochenschrift 1888, No. 38.
86. Deutsche Zeitschrift für Nervenheilkunde I, p. 283 with references to related literature.
87. Cf. my paper in Archiv für Ohrenheilkunde XXXV.
88. Pflügers Archiv. 1882, XXVII, p. 436.
89. Pathologie et traitement de la surdité. Paris, 1883, p. 215.
90. Archiv für Ohrenheilkunde XVI, p. 171, cf. p. 46.
91. Pflügers Archiv. 1882, XXVII, p. 446.
92. Wiener medizinische Presse 1875.
93. Pflügers Archiv. 1882, XXVII, p. 436.
94. Cf. Poggendorfs Annalen. 1857, CI, p. 492; 1859, CVII, p. 653.
95. Arbeiten an der physiologischen Anstalt zu Leipzig, reported by Ludwig. Leipzig, 1872, p. 1.
96. Pflügers Archiv für Physiologie 1881, XXIV.
97. Wiener med. Presse. 1887; see also Gradenigo, Schwartzes Handb.d. Ohrenhk. II, p. 401.
98. Über den Einfluss einer Sinneserregung auf die übrigen Sinnesempfindungen. (Influence of excitation of one sense modality on the other modalities). Pflügers Archiv für Physiologie 1888, XLII, p. 10.
99. See appendix.
100. See Frank, Ohrenheilkunde, 1845, p. 133. The same observation is reported by Gellé (Societié Biolo-

gie. 19 April, 1884. Maladies de l'oreille, 1885, p. 342).

101. Zeitschrift für Ohrenheilkunde 1883, XII, p. 163.
102. Pflüger's Archiv. XXX, p. 153; XXXI, p. 280.
103. Bericht der sächsischen Gesellschaft der Wissenschaften. 1858.
104. S. Funke in Hermanns Handbuch der Physiologie, 1880.
105. Zeitschr.f.Ohrenhk. XII, p. 258.
106. Badische Annalen der Gerichtsarztheikunde. VII, p. 4.
107. Examen chirurgique de sourdsmuets. Paris, 1843.
108. Maladies de l'oreille. 1873, p. 133, 528.
109. Nervenpathologie und Elektrotherapie. 1874, p. 449; Berliner klinische Wochenschrift 1894, No. 31.
110. Naturforscher-Versammlung in Wien. 1894.
111. See Archiv für Ohrenheilkunde XXXVII, p. 272.
112. Tagblatt der Versammlung deutscher Naturforscher und Aerzte. 66. Versammlung II, Th., 2 Hälfte, p. 264.
113. Ohrenheilkunde. 1893, p. 593.
114. Schwartze's Handbuch der Ohrenheilkunde, 1893, II, p. 644; Mygind, Taubstummheit, 1894, Berlin und Leipzig, Verlag Coblenz.
115. 14. Jaresbericht der niederösterreichischen Landes-Taubstummenschule in Wien-Döbling. 1895, p. 79. (Fourteenth annual report of the Lower Austrian School for the Deaf in Vienna-Döbling).
116. See Agramer Zeitung. 10 November, 1893.
117. See also Toynbee, Ohrenheilkunde 1860, translated from English by Moos, 1863, p. 418.
118. 13. Jahresbericht (Annual Report) of the Döbling School for the Deaf, 1893–94, p. 16.
119. Die Krankheiten des Gehörorganes, 1827, p. 37.
120. Richter, Chirurgische Bibliothek. X.
121. Otologischer Congress in Mailand, 1880.
122. Pflügers Archiv für Physiologie 1883, XXXI, p. 287; Archiv für Ohrenheilkunde 1892, XXXIII, p. 186.
123. See Archiv für Ohrenheilkunde XXXIII, p. 197.
124. Ohrenheilkunde 1890, p. 417.
125. Über eine künstliche Gehörverbesserung. Kiel, 1884 Zeitschrift für Ohrenheilkunde XVII, p. 258.
126. British Medical Association in Cork. 1879. See Archiv für Ohrenheilkunde XVI, p. 229.
127. Pflüger's Archiv für Physiologie, XXX, p. 127.
128. Zeitschrift für Ohrenheilkunde XII, p. 121.
129. Wiener klinische Wochenschrift 1894, January, No. 1.
130. Wiener klinische Wochenschrift 1894, No. 1.
131. See appendix, p. 97.